Curbside Consultation
in Fracture Management

49 Clinical Questions

CURBSIDE CONSULTATION IN ORTHOPEDICS
SERIES

SERIES EDITOR, BERNARD R. BACH, JR., MD

Curbside
Consultation
in Fracture Management
49 Clinical Questions

EDITED BY

Walter W. Virkus, MD
Associate Professor
Department of Orthopaedic Surgery
Rush University Medical Center
Chicago, IL

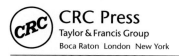

CRC Press
Taylor & Francis Group
Boca Raton London New York

CRC Press is an imprint of the
Taylor & Francis Group, an **informa** business

First published 2008 by SLACK Incorporated

Published 2024 by CRC Press
2385 NW Executive Center Drive, Suite 320, Boca Raton FL 33431

and by CRC Press
4 Park Square, Milton Park, Abingdon, Oxon, OX14 4RN

CRC Press is an imprint of Taylor & Francis Group, LLC

© 2008 Taylor & Francis Group, LLC

Library of Congress Cataloging-in-Publication Data

Curbside consultation in fracture management : 49 clinical questions / edited by Walter W. Virkus.
   p. ; cm.
Includes bibliographical references and index.
ISBN 978-1-55642-829-6 (alk. paper)
1. Fractures--Treatment--Miscellanea. I. Virkus, Walter W.
[DNLM: 1. Fractures, Bone--therapy. WE 180 C975 2008]
RD101.C887 2008
617.1'5--dc22
                                                    2008008706

ISBN: 9781556428296 (pbk)
ISBN: 9781003523512 (ebk)

DOI: 10.1201/9781003523512

Dedication

To my family for their patience and understanding while putting this book together; the residents at Rush, Northwestern, and UIC for their hard work and willingness to learn; and our trauma patients, who always present us with new challenges.

Contents

Acknowledgments

I would like to thank my partner Bernie Bach for asking me to take on this endeavor, Carrie Kotlar, Kim Shigo, and Debra Toulson at SLACK Incorporated for all their hard work and assistance, and my trauma mentors Andy Burgess, MD and David Helfet, MD for all they have done for me and my career.

About the Editor

Walter W. Virkus, MD is an Associate Professor of Orthopaedic Surgery at Rush University Medical Center in Chicago, IL. His practice focuses on orthopedic trauma and orthopedic oncology. He did his residency at the University of Maryland, and trauma fellowships at Shock Trauma in Baltimore, MD and the Hospital for Special Surgery in New York, NY. He then did an oncology fellowship at the University of Florida.

Dr. Virkus is active in research with a special interest in applying trauma techniques to limb preservation in oncology patients. He is very active in resident education and serves as the Associate Program Director for the Rush Orthopaedic Residency.

Contributing Authors

Scott A. Adams, MD, FRCS
Consultant Orthopaedic Trauma Surgeon
Ministry of Defence Hospital Unit (MDHU)
Derriford
Plymouth, UK

Michael T. Archdeacon, MD, MSE
Director, Division of Musculoskeletal
Traumatology
Associate Professor & Vice Chairman,
Department of Orthopaedic Surgery
University of Cincinnati Medical Center
Cincinnati, OH

Timothy Bhattacharyya, MD
Partners Orthopaedic Trauma Service
Massachusetts General Hospital
Brigham and Women's Hospital
Boston, MA

Robert E. Blease, MD
Orthopedic Trauma Fellow
University of Tennessee College of
Medicine-Chattanooga Unit
Chattanooga, TN

Andrew R. Burgess, MD
Academic Chairman, Department of
Orthopaedic Surgery
Director of Trauma, Orthopaedic Faculty
Practice
Orlando Regional Hospital
Orlando, FL
Professor of Orthopaedics
Johns Hopkins University
Baltimore, MD

Mark S. Cohen, MD
Professor
Director, Hand and Elbow Section
Director, Orthopaedic Education
Rush University Medical Center
Chicago, IL

Cory Collinge, MD
Harris Methodist Hospital-Fort Worth
Orthopaedic Specialty Associates
Fort Worth, TX

Dave Dean, DO
Orthopedic Resident
St. Joseph Health Center
Warren, OH

Joseph D. DiCicco, DO
Chief of Orthopedic Surgery
Grandview Hospital
Clinical Professor, Ohio University and
Wright State University
Dayton, OH

Kenneth A. Egol, MD
NYU Hospital for Joint Diseases
Department of Orthopaedic Surgery
New York, NY

John J. Fernandez, MD, FAAOS
Director of Microsurgery
Midwest Orthopaedics at Rush
Assistant Professor of Orthopaedics
Rush University Medical Center
Chicago, IL

Amon T. Ferry, MD
Orthopaedic Resident
Department of Orthopedic Surgery
Rush University Medical Center
Chicago, IL

John C. P. Floyd, MD
Orthopedic Trauma Fellow
Shock Trauma Orthopaedics
University of Maryland Department of
Orthopaedics
Baltimore, MD

Andrew J. Furey, MSc, MD, FRCSC
R Adams Cowley Shock Trauma Center
University of Maryland School of
Medicine
Department of Orthopedics
Baltimore, MD

Rajeev Garapati, MD
Illinois Bone and Joint Institute
Assistant Clinical Professor
University of Illinois at Chicago
Chicago, IL

Michael Garcia, MD
Resident Physician
Loyola University Medical Center
Maywood, IL

Stuart M. Gold, MD
Chief, Fracture Reconstruction Harbor-UCLA
Associate Clinical Professor, UCLA School of Medicine
Director, Orthopaedic Institute
Torrance, CA

Craig Castleman Greene, MD
Traumatology & Sports Medicine
LSUHSC Orthopaedics
Baton Rouge Orthopaedic Clinic
Baton Rouge, LA

Matthew W. Heckler, DO
Orthopedic Surgery Resident
Grandview Hospital
Dayton, OH

Thomas F. Higgins, MD
Assistant Professor, Orthopaedic Trauma
University Orthopaedic Center
University of Utah
Salt Lake City, UT

Micah C. Hobbs, DO
Orthopedic Surgery Resident
Grandview Hospital
Dayton, OH

Matthew L. Jimenez, MD
Illinois Bone and Joint Institute
Morton Grove, IL
Clinical Associate Professor,
Rosalind Franklin University of Medicine and Science
North Chicago, IL

James Kapotas, MD
Division of Orthopedic Surgery
Stroger Cook County Hospital
Chicago, IL

Armen S. Kelikian, MD
Clinical Professor of Orthopedic Surgery
Northwestern University Medical School
Chicago, IL

Najeeb Khan, MD
Resident Physician
McGaw Medical Center
Department of Orthopaedic Surgery
Northwestern University
Chicago, IL

Pradeep Kodali, MD
Resident Physician
McGaw Medical Center
Department of Orthopaedic Surgery
Northwestern University
Chicago, IL

Monica Kogan, MD
Rush University Medical Center
Pediatric Orthopaedics
Chicago, IL

Andrea S. Kramer, MD
Pediatric Orthopaedic Surgeon
Illinois Bone and Joint Institute, LLC
Chicago, IL

Daniel K. Laino, MD
NYU Hospital for Joint Diseases
Department of Orthopaedic Surgery
New York, NY

Gerald J. Lang, MD
Associate Professor of Orthopedic Surgery
University of Wisconsin
Madison, WI

Simon Lee, MD
Rush University Medical Center
Assistant Professor of Orthopaedics
Foot and Ankle Section
Chicago, IL

Johnny L. Lin, MD
Midwest Orthopaedics
Foot and Ankle Specialist
Winfield, IL

Medardo Marota, MD
Orthopedic Resident
Department of Orthopedic Surgery
Rush University Medical Center
Chicago, IL

Michael J. Medvecky, MD
Assistant Professor
Department of Orthopaedics &
Rehabilitation
Yale University School of Medicine
New Haven, CT

Bradley R. Merk, MD
Assistant Professor of Orthopaedic
Surgery
Director of Orthopaedic Trauma
Feinberg School of Medicine
Northwestern University
Chicago, IL

Steven J. Morgan, MD, FACS
Associate Professor
University of Colorado School of Medicine
Department of Orthopaedics
Denver Health Medical Center
Denver, CO

Jason W. Nascone, MD
Assistant Professor
University of Maryland School of
Medicine
Baltimore, MD

Peter J. Nowotarski, MD
Director of Orthopedic Trauma
Associate Professor
University of Tennessee College of
Medicine—Chattanooga Unit
Chattanooga, TN

Robert V. O'Toole, MD
R Adams Cowley Shock Trauma Center
University of Maryland School of
Medicine
Department of Orthopedics
Baltimore, MD

George Partal, MD
Orthopedic Trauma Fellow
Shock Trauma Orthopaedics
University of Maryland Department of
Orthopaedics
Baltimore, MD

Edward A. Perez, MD
Assistant Professor
University of Tennessee/Campbell Clinic
Memphis, TN

Laura Prokuski, MD
Department of Orthopedic Surgery
University of Wisconsin
Madison, WI

Rachel S. Rohde, MD
Orthopaedic Upper Extremity Surgery
Hand and Microvascular Surgery
Weissman, Gitlin, Herkowitz M.D. P.C
Southfield, MI

Anthony G. Sanzone, MD
Associate Director, San Diego Orthopaedic
Trauma Fellowship, OTFS Research &
Education Foundation
Assistant Clinical Professor–Voluntary,
University of California San Diego

John F. Sarwark, MD
Division Head
Division of Pediatric Orthopaedic Surgery
Children's Memorial Hospital
Chicago, IL

Marcus F. Sciadini, MD
Assistant Professor
Shock Trauma Orthopaedics
University of Maryland Department of
Orthopaedics
Baltimore, MD

Blane Sessions, MD
Orthopaedic Resident
LSU Health Sciences Center
New Orleans, LA

Jeffrey M. Smith, MD
Orthopaedic Traumatologist
Orthopaedic Trauma & Fracture Specialists
Medical Corp.
Director, San Diego Orthopaedic Trauma
Fellowship, OTFS Research & Education
Foundation
Assistant Clinical Professor–Voluntary,
University of California San Diego
San Diego, CA

Brian D. Solberg, MD
Director, Orthopaedic Trauma
Cedars Sinai Medical Center
Los Angeles, CA

Anthony T. Sorkin, MD
Director, Orthopedic Traumatology
Rockford Orthopedic Associates, LTD
University of Illinois School of Medicine at
Rockford
Rush University
Chicago, IL

Adam J. Starr, MD
Department of Orthopaedic Surgery
University of Texas Southwestern Medical
Center
Dallas, TX

Michael D. Stover, MD
Fracture Surgeon
Pelvic and Acetabular Reconstruction
Loyola University Medical Center
Maywood, IL

Ishaq Syed, MD
Orthopedic Resident
Department of Orthopedic Surgery
Rush University Medical Center
Chicago, IL

Clifford Turen, MD
R Adams Cowley Shock Trauma Center
University of Maryland School of
Medicine
Department of Orthopaedics
Baltimore, MD

Heather A. Vallier, MD
Associate Professor of Orthopaedic
Surgery
Case Western Reserve University
The MetroHealth System
Cleveland, OH

Robert Vander Griend, MD
Associate Professor
University of Florida
Department of Orthopaedics &
Rehabilitation
Gainesville, FL

Robert W. Wysocki, MD
Orthopedic Resident
Department of Orthopedic Surgery
Rush University Medical Center
Chicago, IL

Bruce H. Ziran, MD
Director of Orthopaedic Trauma
St. Elizabeth Health Center
Associate Professor of Orthopaedic
Surgery
Northeast Ohio Universities College of
Medicine
Rootstown, OH

Introduction

Curbside Consultation in Fracture Management is a unique approach to provide the latest information on the evolving treatment of the trauma patient. The style is casual and designed to be similar to a hallway conversation between colleagues. The questions were chosen to try to span the spectrum of preoperative, operative, and postoperative controversies throughout the skeleton and across all age groups. The questions were answered by practicing, fellowship-trained physicians who are leaders in their field. When possible, current literature was used to support the opinions offered in the questions. When quality literature was lacking, the expert gave his or her opinion on how he or she would handle things in daily practice, as well as reasonable alternatives. Pertinent but not excessive images and references are provided to allow the book to be used as a quick reference for the clinical problems presented. The short format also allowed the books to be created much faster than larger textbooks, allowing the material to be up-to-date at publication.

Foreword

When Dr. Virkus asked me to write a foreword on *Curbside Consultation in Fracture Management: 49 Clinical Questions,* I was, obviously, very honored but not sure what to expect. I was very pleasantly surprised: not only is this a good idea, ie, answering the oft-asked questions we all routinely face emergently, but in a most concise and informative manner, and all by multiple orthopaedic trauma surgeons with experience. With 49 such questions posed, the spectrum covered is huge—from the clavicle to the toes, from kids to the elderly, from low to high energy and even polytrauma patients.

There is no shortage of orthopaedic information available, even immediate access through the internet, so why this?

This is the only attempt, to my knowledge, that focuses on and answers only the pertinent dilemma of the moment, without having to spend a lot of time gleaning such information indirectly from the internet, articles, books, etc.

Dr. Virkus is to be congratulated on a very good idea, and he and his co-authors on making it happen in a very user-friendly manner. Clearly, *Curbside Consultation in Fracture Management* is an excellent resource for all who treat fractures and take ER call—but especially the younger generation with less experience such as residents, fellows, and junior staff. This will definitely become a useful resource for my own residents and fellows.

David L. Helfet, MD
Professor of Orthopaedic Surgery
Weill Medical College of Cornell University
Director, Orthopaedic Trauma Service
Hospital for Special Surgery/New York-Presbyterian Hospital
New York, NY

SECTION I

UPPER EXTREMITIES

I Have a 50-Year-Old Male With a Surgical Neck Humerus Fracture in His Dominant Arm. Should I Operate on Him?

James Kapotas, MD

When dealing with a humeral neck fracture, you must determine if it is an isolated fracture. This requires you to rule out an open injury, nerve or vessel injury, or associated fracture. There should be an anterior-posterior (AP) in the scapular plane, a Y-lateral and an axillary lateral radiograph in order to rule out a dislocation, a tuberosity fracture, or head-splitting fracture. If you are unable to obtain good plain films, consider a CT scan. Once you are confident that it is an isolated fracture, you can then decide if surgery is necessary.

Most isolated surgical neck fractures are minimally displaced and do not need an operation. Minimally displaced fractures include those with less than 1 cm of displacement and less than 45 degrees of angulation. Minimally displaced fractures can be treated in a sling and range of motion exercises started when the patient is comfortable, usually around 2 to 3 weeks.[1]

Displaced fractures require an operation. You cannot perform a closed reduction on a proximal humerus fracture and hold it in a sling; you need some kind of fixation. Your choices include closed reduction and percutaneous pinning, open reduction and internal fixation with a locked proximal humerus plate, or closed or open reduction and intramedullary nailing with a nail that allows screws or a blade to lock to the nail. The choice of technique depends on the ability to reduce the fracture closed, the fracture pattern, the quality of the bone, and surgeon's comfort. It is important to explain to the patient the different techniques available and be prepared in the operating room to make changes. Make sure you have all the equipment ready in case you have to change to a different type of fixation.

My first choice for isolated proximal humerus fractures is closed reduction and percutaneous pinning. I use this technique when there is no comminution or metaphyseal extension and I am able to close reduce the fracture. I place the patient supine with the arm off the side of the table. The fluoroscopy machine comes in from the head of the table. The reduction maneuver is usually traction, abduction of the shoulder, and manipulating the shaft posteriorly to align with the head.[2] Once the fracture is reduced, I then place four terminally threaded pins (2.5 or 2.8 mm) from the lateral aspect of the shaft into the humeral head. The first pin placed is usually the most inferior on the shaft so that the pin is directed toward the most inferior and central part of the head. The three other pins are then place proximal to this pin laterally on the shaft and placed into the head so that there is one anterior, one posterior, and one superior. Make sure there is about a 1-cm space between each pin laterally on the shaft, otherwise you can create a fracture of the lateral cortex. The reduction is then checked with fluoroscopy with an AP view and axillary lateral view. The pins are then cut short, so that they are under the skin. Postoperation, the arm is left in a sling and no shoulder motion is started. The patient can do elbow, hand, and wrist exercises. The pins are removed in the OR at 4 weeks and then the patient can begin pendulum exercises.

If I am unable to reduce the fracture, bone quality is poor, or there is comminution at the fracture site, I will then proceed with open reduction and internal fixation with a locked proximal humeral plate (Figure 1-1).[3] The patient is placed in a beach chair position with a bump under the shoulder. The fluoroscopy machine is located on the opposite side of the table and perpendicular to the table. I approach the fracture through a deltopectoral interval. The fracture is reduced and held with k-wires. The fracture reduction and plate position is then confirmed with fluoroscopy. The plate should be lateral to the biceps tendon, 1-cm distal to the tip of the greater tuberosity so that it does not impinge with abduction of the shoulder, and centered on the humeral shaft. The most distal and most proximal humeral head screws are appropriately placed. Range of motion is begun immediately postop.

In cases where there is metaphyseal/diaphyseal extension, I prefer to fix the fracture with an intramedullary nail with screws or a blade that lock into the nail proximally. The advantage of a nail in this case is less dissection and a quicker recovery. The patient is placed in a floppy lateral position on a radiolucent table. The fluoroscopy machine is placed on the opposite side of the table and perpendicular to the table. In cases where the fracture can be reduced closed, I use a deltoid split incision. In cases where there needs to be an open reduction, I use a delto-pectoral approach. It is important to start the nail appropriately. Make an incision through the rotator cuff just posterior to the bicipital groove and midline on the lateral view. Lock the nail proximally and distally. It is important to close the rotator cuff incision. Range of motion is begun immediately postop.

References

1. Rowles D, McGrory J. Percutaneous pinning of the proximal part of the humerus: an anatomic study. *J Bone Joint Surg Am.* 2001;83-A:1695-1699.
2. Jaberg H, Warner JJ, Jakob RP. Percutaneous stabilization of unstable fractures of the humerus. *J Bone Joint Surg Am.* 1992;74-A:508-515.

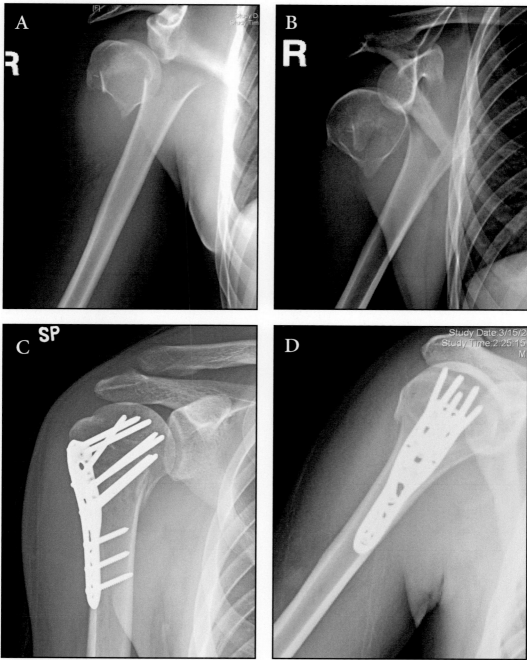

Figure 1-1. AP (A) and lateral (B) radiograph of a displaced surgical neck fracture. Postoperative AP (C) and lateral (D) radiographs demonstrate reduction with a locking plate.

3. Edwards S, et al. Two part surgical neck fracture of the proximal part of the humerus: a biomechanical evaluation of two fixation techniques. *J Bone Joint Surg Am.* 2006;88-A:2258-2264.

WHAT APPROACH SHOULD I USE FOR PLATING A HUMERAL SHAFT FRACTURE IN A MULTIPLE TRAUMA PATIENT?

Adam J. Starr, MD

The choice of surgical approach for humeral shaft fractures in a patient with multiple injuries depends on several factors. The patient's condition, the fracture anatomy, and the surgical team all have an impact on the selection of a surgical exposure.

First, consider the condition of the patient. Humeral fracture repair can be bloody—can the patient tolerate blood loss? If the patient is unstable, it may best to postpone humeral repair. If the patient is able to tolerate surgery, the patient's status and ability to tolerate supine, lateral, or prone positioning may change your selected approach.

Next, think about what the fracture looks like. Will you need an extensile exposure to control it?

Finally, how much help do you have? If I am operating alone, I may select an approach that does not require an assistant to hold the arm.

My preferred exposure is a posterior approach that mobilizes the triceps muscle, shifting it medially, as described by Gerwin et al[1] (Figure 2-1). I like this approach because it offers excellent access to the humerus, it is friendly to the soft tissues (muscles are mobilized rather than cut), and it leaves a cosmetically acceptable scar. Patients tend to like it better than the anterolateral incision.[2,3]

This exposure requires a fairly long incision and large dissection of the posterior arm. However, the scar is on the back of the arm and so it is cosmetically acceptable—far more so than the easily noticeable anterolateral incision—and the extensive dissection of the triceps muscle does little damage to the tissues. The triceps is spared, not split, and so active function is possible immediately after fixation.

If a surgical assistant is available, the procedure can be done with the patient in a supine position, which is generally preferable for multiply injured patients. The surgeon stands on the injured side while the assistant holds the arm draped across the patient's chest. If no assistant is available, the patient should be placed in a lateral decubitus

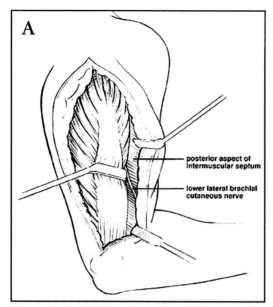

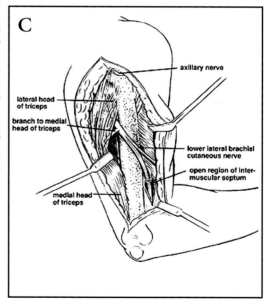

Figure 2-1. (A) The lower brachial cutaneous nerve, which branches off of the radial nerve, is identified along the posterior aspect of the intermuscular septum. (B) The intermuscular septum is divided deep to the lower lateral brachial cutaneous nerve for 3 cm to expose the radial nerve distally. (C) Mobilization of the triceps muscle allows exposure of the posterior humeral shaft. (Reprinted with permission from Gerwin M, Hotchkiss R, Weiland A. Alternative operative exposures of the posterior aspect of the humeral diaphysis with reference to the radial nerve. *J Bone Joint Surg.* 1996;78-A:1690-1695.)

position and the injured arm is propped on a bolster. (If no assistant is available, and the patient cannot be positioned laterally due to pulmonary or other issues, a different approach should be chosen.)

A few tips will make this approach easier. First, make a long incision. Long flaps make retraction easier and less damaging. The scar will be on the posterior arm, and will not be noticeable, so incision length should not be a concern.

Next, be sure to approach the humerus first distally—where it is easiest to find. The illustrations in the article by Gerwin et al[1] show the incision extending to a point a few centimeters proximal to the olecranon. I do it differently. I always carry the incision to the tip of the olecranon so that I have ready access to the distal humerus. Once you've made your skin incision, elevate full thickness skin flaps to expose the triceps fascia. This will make it easy to see the epicondylar ridges of the distal humerus. There are no nerves or vessels lying over the lateral epicondyle. This gives you a free shot at the bone, so you can find it quickly and safely, without struggling. It is safe to dissect down on the lateral epicondyle, elevating the triceps posteriorly. This elevation quickly and safely exposes the underlying distal humerus. Once you've elevated the distal triceps, place a retractor under the muscle and incise the posterior elbow joint capsule. This allows access to the olecranon fossa and improves visualization.

You can carry the dissection proximally by reflecting the triceps muscle belly away from the lateral intermuscular septum of the arm. Begin from the lateral edge of the triceps and roll the muscle up medially, sweeping it away from the septum. The septum will lead you right over to the shaft of the humerus. This is easiest with an elevator. The attachments to the fascia are flimsy and come off easily. Take care not to perforate the fascia itself, as the fascia is your guide to staying on the humerus. If you rip through the fascia, it is easy to wind up on the anterior aspect of the humerus, which is dangerous. Pointed retractors are useful for holding the muscle out of the way as you move proximally.

Dissection near the mid-portion of the humerus often becomes tedious because of concerns about damaging the radial nerve. Surgical textbooks (and Gerwin et al's article[1]) sometimes suggest finding small sensory branches of the nerve distally in order to trace them back and find the radial nerve. My experience has been that this is not worthwhile. Small nerves are not always visible because of fracture hematoma or swelling. The safest thing to do is carefully approach the mid-portion of the humerus from both the proximal and distal to find the nerve and protect it.

When I have completed exposure of the distal third of the humerus, I turn my attention proximally. By elevating full thickness skin flaps, it is easy to see the interval between the deltoid and triceps muscles. The muscles will be swollen and distended with blood from the fracture, but the muscle fibers are oriented differently—it is simple to find the correct plane, as long as your skin incision is long enough. The plane between the two is developed down to the humerus using an elevator. The radial nerve and profunda brachii artery lie medial to the origin of the lateral head of the triceps, so it is safe to elevate the triceps muscle medially, while retracting the deltoid laterally. This dissection allows for access to the proximal one-third of the humeral shaft (see Figure 2-1C). Proximal dissection is limited by the axillary nerve, which crosses the field transversely, but digital access to the shoulder joint capsule is possible.

The ability to access the proximal and distal portions of the humerus is a main strength of this exposure. It will make reduction and internal fixation easier, as well as provide superior access to the humeral shaft.

Once you have access to the proximal and distal portions of the humerus, dissection should be carried toward the bone's mid-section, where the radial nerve crosses and where the fracture commonly lies. I typically work a little bit from one direction, then a little bit from the other until I am sure of the nerve's location.

The nerve is always found in a layer of fat. Small sensory branches are usually visible heading distally, but these are not dependable markers of the nerve's location. They may be hidden by hematoma or swelling. The radial nerve must be handled carefully. It is tethered proximally by the triangular interval, and distally by the intermuscular septum.

It will not tolerate excessive retraction, but the broad exposure using this approach makes identification of the nerve easy. Thus, neuropraxia following this approach is rare.

Although Gerwin et al's illustration shows the nerve being left lying adjacent to the humerus, dissected completely free from the triceps muscle belly, I usually try to leave the nerve attached to the triceps as much as possible, and work under it. It will be necessary to elevate the nerve from the bone to place the plate for fracture repair, so I advise leaving some of the local tissue attachments intact.

Once reduction and fixation are complete, the retractors are removed and the triceps muscle falls back into place. The muscle is usually too swollen to permit closure of the triceps fascia, but the skin can be closed easily in layers.

Preservation of the triceps is another main strength of this approach. The muscle is left intact and, in my experience, recovers well after surgery. Patients usually are able to begin active extension of the elbow very quickly.

References

1. Gerwin M, Hotchkiss R, Weiland A. Alternative operative exposures of the posterior aspect of the humeral diaphysis with reference to the radial nerve. *J Bone Joint Surg.* 1996;78-A:1690-1695.
2. Hoppenfeld S, de Boer P. *Surgical Exposures in Orthopaedics. The Anatomic Approach.* Philadelphia, PA: Lippincott Williams and Wilkins; 2003.
3. Henry AK. *Extensile Exposure.* 2nd ed. Edinburgh: Churchill Livingstone; 1973.

HOW WOULD YOU MANAGE A RADIAL NERVE PALSY ASSOCIATED WITH A HUMERAL SHAFT FRACTURE IN THE DOMINANT ARM OF A 25-YEAR-OLD?

Laura Prokuski, MD

The radial nerve has an intricate relationship with the humerus. From its origin in the posterior cord of the brachial plexus, the radial nerve enters the triangular interval with the profunda brachii artery, bounded by long and lateral heads of the triceps and the teres major. It is closely associated with the shaft of the humerus and is found adjacent to the mid-portion of the bone in the spiral grove. The nerve traverses the intermuscular septum, and is found distally between the brachialis and the brachioradialis.

With the humerus and radial nerve in such close proximity, it seems reasonable that a force applied to the arm large enough to fracture the humerus may also injure the radial nerve. Radial nerve palsy occurs in 8.5% to 12% of humerus fractures. Middle and middle-distal fractures have a higher association with radial nerve palsy, as do transverse and spiral patterns of fracture.[1,2]

In the patient who presents with a closed humerus fracture and a radial nerve palsy, the radial nerve is usually intact and the prognosis for complete or near complete recovery is good.[3] Laceration of the radial nerve in association with a closed diaphyseal fracture of the humerus is unusual, even when the fracture is the result of a high energy injury mechanism.[3,4] Radial nerve recovery is similar whether observation or early exploration is utilized.[5]

A patient may have a closed humeral fracture with radial nerve initially working, but a palsy ensues after reduction, splinting, or a period of observation (secondary palsy). Since closed injuries are usually associated with structurally intact nerves, and intact nerves nearly always recover, there is no support for radial nerve exploration in secondary palsies.[3] The recovery rate after observing primary nerve palsy (88.6%) and secondary nerve palsy (93%) is similar.[1]

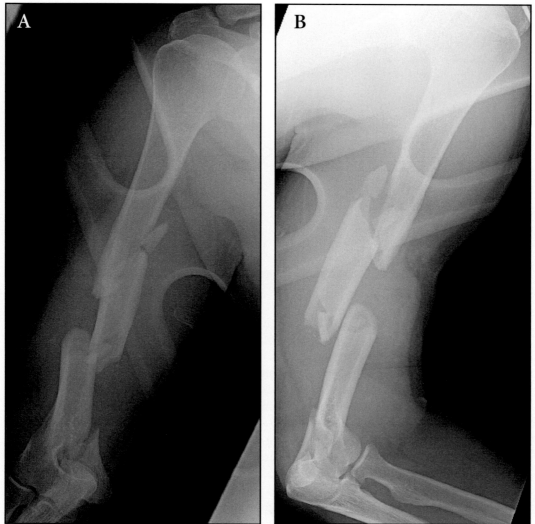

Figure 3-1. Anterior-posterior (A) and lateral (B) views of a segmental open humerus fracture with an associated radial nerve palsy.

In closed humerus fractures, characteristics of the patient, the limb, and the injury influence whether operative stabilization or fracture brace treatment will be utilized to treat the skeletal injury. I don't think radial nerve palsy alone is an indication for surgical treatment of a humerus fracture that would otherwise be treated with a fracture brace.

Operative treatment is necessary in open humerus fractures to debride the exposed bone and to perform skeletal stabilization. Radial nerve disruption is strongly associated with open fracture of the humerus, and exploration of the nerve is recommended.[3,4] Ring et al[3] demonstrated that radial nerve disruption in high energy open humerus fractures is rarely a sharp laceration. Often the nerve has been crushed or avulsed.[3]

Characteristics of the open wound and characteristics of the humerus fracture are factors that determine which surgical approach will be used to accomplish debridement,

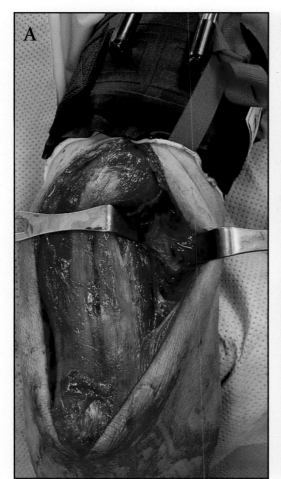 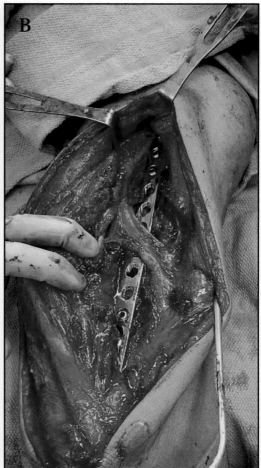

Figure 3-2. (A) Intraoperative photograph of a posterior approach to the humerus. The radial nerve is located on the posterior aspect of the intermuscular septum on the lateral side of the arm, between the retractors. The triceps is retracted medially. (B) Intraoperative photograph demonstrates the humerus has been exposed, debrided, and stabilized with a plate. The triceps is retracted medially. The radial nerve has been explored and is structurally intact. The radial nerve is demonstrated to be superficial to the plate.

skeletal stabilization, and radial nerve exploration. These tasks can be accomplished through a posterior triceps-splitting, posterior triceps-sparing, lateral, or an anterior approach. Direct repair or grafting of a disrupted radial nerve can be performed after skeletal stabilization. The return of radial nerve function in this situation is variable, and likely depends on the severity of the structural damage to the nerve.[3,4]

During observation of a radial nerve palsy, I place the wrist in a simple splint. Active finger and thumb flexion are encouraged, and passive stretching should be performed routinely. Splinting of the fingers in extension at rest may be helpful in some patients.

Since most radial nerve injuries associated with a closed fracture recover, at what point should further investigation or procedures be performed for those with no recovery? The first signs of radial nerve recovery can take longer than 6 months and complete recovery

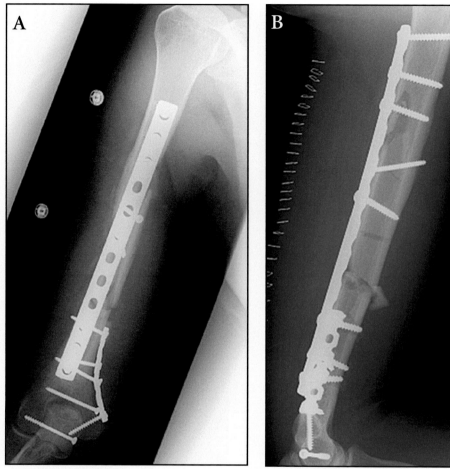

Figure 3-3. Anteriorposterior (A) and lateral (B) views of the humerus after skeletal stabilization. The triceps sparing posterior approach provides nearly full access to the humerus and the radial nerve.

can take 2 years or more.[3,5] Shao et al[1] reported the mean time to the onset of spontaneous recovery was 7.3 weeks, which may indicate the minimum waiting time before exploration. The optimal time of observation before intervention has been debated, but no clear answer is universally supported.

Nerve conduction velocities and electromyography are often used to look for radial nerve recovery when none is clinically apparent. Negative electrical studies, however, cannot distinguish between a severed nerve and a nonfunctioning intact nerve.[3] Results from electrical studies parallel clinical findings. Electrical signs of recovery occur no more than a month before recovery becomes apparent clinically.[3,5] Therefore, I usually don't order electrical studies unless the patient is 4 to 6 months from injury with no sign of recovery.

Nerve exploration, neurolysis, and grafting have been performed in attempts to restore radial nerve function. Variation exists in the reported time thresholds for exploration

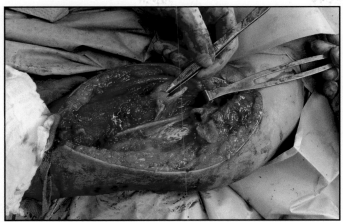

Figure 3-4. Intraoperative photograph of radial nerve exploration through an anterior approach to the humerus. The radial nerve is demonstrated on the lateral aspect of the arm. It is localized distally between the brachialis and brachioradialis, then dissected proximally. The humerus fragments are retracted anteriorly, exposing the more proximal portion of the radial nerve. The nerve has traumatic laceration of a few fascicles at the fracture site.

and recovery rates.[1] Nerve exploration for possible grafting may be most appropriate in patients who can tolerate a wrist brace, long recovery periods, and an uncertain outcome.[3] I reserve this for patients 6 to 12 months from injury with no signs of recovery.

For patients where radial nerve function has not recovered, tendon transfers provide predictably good restoration of hand function, but cannot restore fine independent finger extension.[3] Recommendations vary on the clinical situations that should lead to tendon transfers. Persistent palsy after an extended recovery period, persistent palsy after neurolysis or grafting, and patients who want rapid return of function or limited surgical intervention are reasonable candidates for tendon transfers. Timing is usually at least a year from injury to allow for possible recovery.

References

1. Shao YC, Harwood P, Grotz MRW, Limb D, Giannoudis PV. Radial nerve palsy associated with fractures of the humerus. a systematic review. *J Bone Joint Surg.* 2005;87B:1647-1652.
2. Ekholm R, Adami J, Tidermark J, Hansson K, Tornkvist H, Ponzer S. Fractures of the shaft of the humerus. an epidemiological study of 401 fractures. *J Bone Joint Surg.* 2006;88B:1469-1473.
3. Ring D, Chin K, Jupiter JB. Radial nerve palsy associated with high-energy humeral shaft fractures. *J Hand Surg.* 2004;29:144-147.
4. Fister RJ, Swiontkowski MF, Bach AW, Sack JT. Radial nerve palsy caused by open humeral shaft fractures. *J Hand Surg.* 1993;18A:121-124.
5. Shah JJ, Bhatti NA. Radial nerve paralysis associated with fractures of the humerus: a review of 62 cases. *Clin Orthop.* 1983;172:171-176.

ON WHICH CLAVICLE FRACTURES DO YOU OPERATE?

Brian D. Solberg, MD

Clavicle fractures are common injuries typically seen in active, young adults and are usually a result of direct trauma to the shoulder region. Conservative management using a sling or figure of 8 brace has been the mainstay of treatment.[1,2] Reported rates of malunion and nonunion in the literature have been low and possibly under-reported in the general population.[3] Recent data from a large prospective multicenter trial demonstrated higher rates of union, higher DASH scores, and lower rates of malunion, nonunion, and complications in displaced clavicular shaft fractures treated with open reduction and internal fixation (ORIF) using a cephelad plate.[4,5]

The data still supports conservative management for a vast majority of clavicle fractures, however there is a subset that has better overall outcomes with operative management. I treat fractures with more than 1.5 cm of medialization of the acromioclavicular (AC) joint, more than 1 cm diastasis between fragment ends, open fractures, or fractures in which the proximal fragment punctures the clavi-pectoral fascia (Figure 4-1) with open repair. Medialization of the shoulder produces a fairly noticeable asymmetry of the shoulder contour on the involved side and the distance from the manubrial notch to the AC joint or lateral acromion can be measured. Likewise, a subcutaneous position of the proximal fragment often produces a puckering of the skin at the end of the proximal fragment with the sharp end of the fracture palpable in the subcutaneous position.

Radiographically, clavicular fractures are easily diagnosed; however, it is difficult to obtain a true lateral of the shaft fragment, making assessment of length problematic from the radiographs alone. With higher energy fractures, comminution will often occur, producing a vertical intercalary fragment that helps to quantify the amount of displacement (Figure 4-2). Although concomitant AC joint injury and/or dislocation is uncommon with displaced clavicular shaft fractures, radiographs should include AC and sternoclavicular (SC) joints to rule out involvement and/or asymmetry. Postoperative radiographs must

Figure 4-1. AP radiograph of a displaced clavicular shaft fracture in which the proximal fragment has perforated the clavi-pectoral fascia and is sitting in a subcutaneous position.

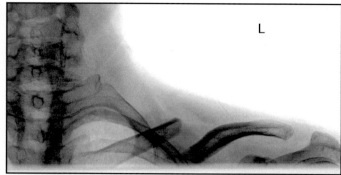

Figure 4-2. High energy clavicular shaft fracture with intercalary segment vertically oriented.

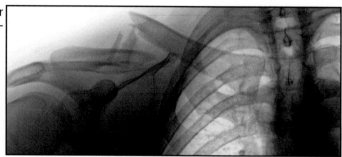

Figure 4-3. Grade II AC joint separation found on the postoperative radiograph. The separation was not evident on preop radiographs.

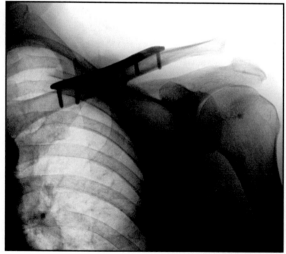

also include the AC joint as described cases of missed AC dislocation have been found on postop radiographs even though the preop radiograph is often negative (Figure 4-3).

Repair of the fracture is done with the patient in a beach chair position, arm draped free, and a small roll between the scapulae. Tilting the head to the contralateral side is helpful to place the medial screws in the plate. Incision over the subcutaneous border of the clavicle is carried in a curvilinear fashion. The skin in this area is pliable and typically skin edges can be mobilized in either direction for several centimeters, allowing the skin

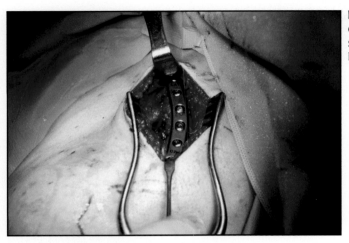

Figure 4-4. Skin edges are typically pliable, allowing skin incisions to be shorter than the plate length.

incisions to be smaller than the plate length in many cases (Figure 4-4). Preservation of the crossing supra-clavicular nerve branches lessens the amount of postoperative cutaneous numbness but has not been shown to have an impact on DASH scores or outcomes. Autogenous bone graft is unnecessary for acute fractures except in cases with segmental defects or bone loss.

Fixation of the fracture typically is performed with small and mini-fragment implants. If the fracture has a long oblique pattern or large intercalary segment, I prefer to place two interfragmentary lag screws to provisionally hold the fracture. Mini-fragment (2.0-mm) screws are more applicable for this purpose because small fragment (3.5-mm) screws are generally too large and will often split the fragment. Plate fixation is generally carried out using small fragment plates or precontoured plates. Reconstruction plates are often adequate for women and smaller adults but are problematic in adult males with bending and/or breakage reported (Figure 4-5). Precontoured plates are thicker with a higher load-to-failure strength, making them a better alternative in men. Standard small fragment implants can also be used but require intraoperative bending, which prolongs the surgical procedure and may weaken the plate. Other implants such as one-third or one-fourth tubular plates lack bending and rotational strength and are not recommended. Intraoperative radiographs should be obtained before leaving the operating room to rule out pneumothorax and to double check screw length.

Postoperatively, patients are allowed range of motion to tolerance and generally regain 90% to 95% of motion within the first 2 weeks of surgery. Lifting for the first 6 weeks is restricted to 5 lbs and contact sports are restricted for the first 3 months. Plate irritation is a common problem, especially in women or thin patients, and many request plate removal in the future. Counseling patients about this potential prior to surgery is important and has a small effect of patient satisfaction and outcomes. Plate removal can be safely carried out at 6 to 9 months postsurgery and the rate of refracture through the screw holes is low (1% to 4%).

Figure 4-5. Failure of 3.5 mm reconstruction plate in a young male patient.

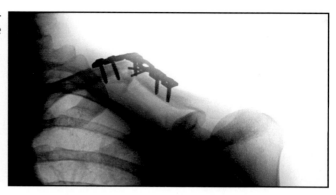

References

1. Neer CS. Non union of the clavicle. *JAMA.* 1960;172:1006-1011.
2. Rowe CR. An atlas of anatomy and treatment of midclavicular fractures. *Clin Orthop Relat Res.* 1968;58:29-42.
3. Robinson CM, Court-Brown CM, McQueen MM, Wakefield AE. Estimating the risk of nonunion following nonoperative treatment of a clavicular fracture. *J Bone Joint Surg Am.* 2004;86:1359-1365.
4. Zlowodzki M, Zelle BA, Cole PA, Jeray K, McKee MD; Evidence-Based Orthopaedic Trauma Working Group. Treatment of midshaft clavicle fractures: systemic review of 2144 fractures: on behalf of the Evidence-Based Orthopaedic Trauma Working Group. *J Orthop Trauma.* 2005;19:504-507.
5. Canadian Orthopaedic Trauma Society. Nonoperative treatment compared with plate fixation of displaced midshaft clavicular fracture: a multicenter randomized clinical trial. *J Bone Joint Surg Am.* 2007;89:1-10.

WHAT IS YOUR POSTOPERATIVE AND REHABILITATIVE PROTOCOL FOR DISTAL HUMERAL FRACTURES?

Amon T. Ferry, MD
Mark S. Cohen, MD

Prior to the use of contemporary surgical techniques and aggressive postoperative protocols, operative fixation of intra-articular distal humerus fractures was associated with poor functional outcomes largely due to inadequate fixation or motion loss. The goal of operative treatment is an anatomic reduction of the articular surface and creation of a stable construct that will allow early mobilization. Prolonged immobilization of more than approximately 3 weeks following operative fixation may lead to a loss in functional range of motion.[1,2] Flexion and extension deficits are most commonly encountered following ORIF (open reduction and internal fixation) of distal humerus fractures; deficits in pronation and supination of the forearm, however, are rare. In order to maintain a functional extremity, at least 100 degrees of arc at the ulnohumeral joint is required, from approximately 30 to 130°. Because the function of the elbow is to position the hand in space, loss of motion at this joint is not well-tolerated and an aggressive postoperative protocol is critical to an acceptable outcome.

Postoperative Protocol

We prefer operative fixation of distal humerus fractures via a posterior approach utilizing an olecranon osteotomy to visualize the articular surface in the majority of cases. Triceps "sparing" approaches are available that involve detachment of the triceps from the ulna, but these can lead to triceps weakness.

Immediately following surgery, we place the arm into a well-padded long-arm posterior mold splint (Table 5-1). Cryotherapy (ice application) and elevation are initiated in the recovery room and continued after discharge for the first 3 to 4 postoperative days.

> ## Table 5-1
> ## Postoperative Protocol Following ORIF of a Distal Humerus Fracture
>
> | *Postoperative Week* | *Activity* |
> | --- | --- |
> | 1 | • Immobilized in postop splint |
> | 2 to 6 | • Removable orthoplast splint during the day, extension splint at night
• PROM and AAROM initiated, progression to AROM |
> | 6 to 10 | • Aggressive AROM, no strengthening |
> | >10 | • Muscle strengthening, dynamic splint if needed |
>
> PROM = passive range of motion; AROM = active range of motion; AAROM = active assisted ROM

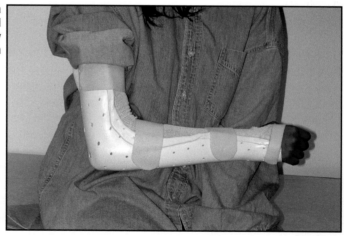

Figure 5-1. Photograph of a patient wearing a custom-molded Othoplast splint with the elbow at 90° of flexion and the wrist in neutral rotation.

The patient is typically seen approximately 1 week after surgery at which time the splint is removed, wounds are evaluated, and radiographs are taken. A removable, custom fitted long-arm Orthoplast (Johnson and Johnson, New Brunswick, NJ) splint is molded to include the wrist with the elbow at 90° (Figure 5-1). Occupational therapy is initiated at this time. This involves edema control including the use of a compression sleeve, education, and hourly exercise out of the splint (Figure 5-2). Formal therapy sessions are also scheduled 2 to 3 times per week. Initially, rehabilitation focuses on active and active assisted range of motion. Gentle passive motion is initially allowed under therapy supervision only. At no time is vigorous manipulation used.

If a patient has difficulty recovering elbow extension, a night Orthoplast splint is fashioned in maximum extension. This splint is adjusted as elbow extension improves. Loading and strengthening are not permitted until there is evidence of bony healing, typically at approximately 2 to 3 months. Office visits are maintained every 2 to 4 weeks

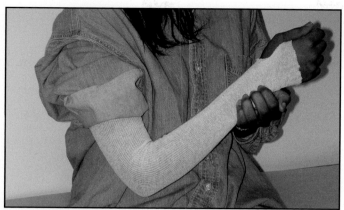

Figure 5-2. Photograph of a patient wearing an edema control sleeve while practicing active AAROM exercises.

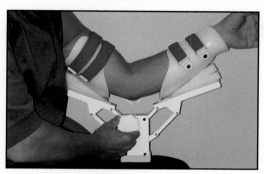

Figure 5-3. Photograph of a patient using a patient-adjusted static splint.

during this time. In cases of prolonged stiffness where there is a plateau in motion, patient-adjusted static splints can be utilized once union has occurred (Figure 5-3). These braces use the principles of passive-progressive stretch and are only required 2 to 3 times per day for approximately 30 minutes.

Stable internal fixation and early mobilization after operative fixation of distal humerus fractures yields predictably favorable results in most patients. Recent advances in implant technology as well as a better understanding of optimal plate osteosynthesis techniques have led to improved functional results after operative treatment.[3-5] Early mobilization following operative fixation of distal humerus fractures is therefore critical to prevent postoperative arthrofibrosis and the maintenance of a functional range of motion.

Postoperative stiffness is typically due to soft tissue contractures, adhesions, and bony impingement. An extension deficit may result from anterior capsular contracture or thickening, adhesions formed between the brachialis and the humerus, and/or bony and soft tissue overgrowth in the olecranon fossa. Similarly, flexion may be blocked if the triceps and posterior capsule become adherent to the humerus, and/or the concavity of the coronoid and radial fossae may become blocked with soft tissue and bony overgrowth. Patients with a greater than 25 to 30 degrees of flexion contracture and/or less than 100 to 115 degrees of flexion who fail appropriate conservative treatment may be candidates for an elbow release procedure. Operative release should be delayed until at least 4 months after ORIF to allow sufficient time for postoperative inflammation to resolve. It must also be emphasized that unless patients are motivated and compliant with the demanding protocol, they are not candidates for elbow release.

References

1. McKee M, Jupiter J. *Fractures of the Distal Humerus*. 3rd ed. Philadelphia, PA: Elsevier; 2003.
2. Waddell JP, Hatch J, Richards R. Supracondylar fractures of the humerus—results of surgical treatment. *J Trauma*. 1988;28:1615-1621.
3. Letsch R, Schmit-Neuerburg KP, Sturmer KM, et al. Intraarticular fractures of the distal humerus. Surgical treatment and results. *Clin Orthop Relat Res*. 1989:238-244.
4. Jupiter JB, Neff U, Holzach P, et al. Intercondylar fractures of the humerus. An operative approach. *J Bone Joint Surg Am*. 1985;67:226-239.
5. Gabel GT, Hanson G, Bennett JB, et al. Intraarticular fractures of the distal humerus in the adult. *Clin Orthop Relat Res*. 1987:99-108.

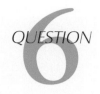

I Have a 4-Year-Old Who Fell Off the Monkey Bars With a Swollen Elbow and a Fat Pad Sign. If the X-rays are Normal, Is Additional Evaluation Needed?

Monica Kogan, MD

Fractures about the elbow account for 5% to 10% of all fractures in children. Supracondylar humerus fractures are the most common, accounting for 50% to 70%[1]; however, fractures of the radial head/neck, proximal ulna, medial and lateral condyles/epicondyles all present with swelling and pain about the elbow. Depending on the severity, the child may present to the emergency department with a displaced fracture the same day or even a day later with nondisplaced or minimally displaced fractures.

Typically, fractures that are displaced will have an obvious deformity and be extremely swollen. It can be more difficult to identify the nondisplaced fracture that presents with swelling and pain, without obvious deformity, as these fractures may not be obvious on radiographs.

A child who presents after a fall with a swollen elbow should have a thorough physical examination and history. Palpation of the medial and lateral epicondyles, olecranon, radial head, proximal ulna, and distal radius and ulna should be performed. Neurovascular status should be evaluated, as well as range of motion, if possible.

Radiographs should always be obtained and should include an anterior posterior, lateral, and an oblique view of the elbow. The radiographs should be evaluated to assure the anterior humeral line aligns with the middle third of the capitellum, the radial head aligns with the capitellum, and be assessed for any fracture lines and presence of a posterior fat pad sign (Figure 6-1).

Figure 6-1. A lateral radiograph of the elbow in a 6-year-old boy who fell on his arm. The radiograph demonstrates the posterior fat pad sign just posterior to the olecranon fossa.

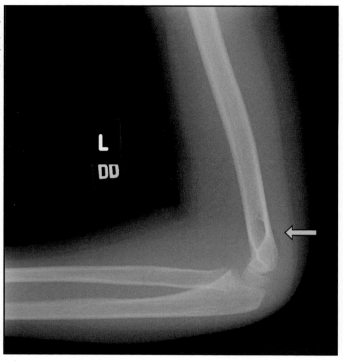

Fractures about the elbow in children may be difficult to identify radiographically because the elbow ossifies at different ages. The capitellum ossifies first at around 1 to 2 years of age and the lateral condyle ossifies last at around age 11 to 12. Because of this, a fracture may be present, although it cannot be identified because it is located in an unossified part of the elbow, and therefore is not visible on radiographs.

At times, the only abnormality seen on the radiographs is a posterior fat pad sign. The posterior fat pad sign indicates that there is bleeding within the joint and that a fracture is present. The posterior fat pad is normally pressed into the olecranon fossa by the triceps and anconeus and is invisible on a true lateral radiograph in a normal elbow flexed 90°. When a fracture is present, the hemarthrosis causes distention of the joint capsule and displacement of the fat pad. The anterior fat pad is considered normal and should not be confused with any pathology present in the elbow. With a fracture however, the anterior fat pad may be displaced more superiorly and anteriorly than normal.[2]

In one study, 76% of children who presented with a swollen elbow, pain, and a positive posterior fat pad sign were found to have fractures identified on follow-up radiographs. The most common fractures were supracondylar humerus fractures, followed by proximal ulna fractures, lateral condyle fractures, and fractures of the radial neck.[3]

When a child presents with a history of a fall, has a swollen, painful elbow, and a posterior fat pad sign, I place the child in a cast for a period of 3 weeks for a "presumed fracture" or occult elbow fracture. I do not perform any further workup such as an MRI, CT scan, or bone scan. These studies are costly, often require sedation, and most likely do not change the child's management. There have been studies that have used MRI to evaluate the presence of fractures in patients with clinical pictures of a fracture but with only a posterior fat pad sign identified on radiographs.[4] These studies revealed that there was no change in the management of the pediatric population. One study that used MRI reported all patients with a posterior fat pad sign had an abnormal MRI, confirming that the posterior fat pad is an adequate indicator of trauma to the elbow.

Young children typically do not know the concept of secondary gain or faking pain. When a child is not moving his or her elbow, it typically is because he or she is experiencing a lot of discomfort and most likely has a fracture. Immobilizing a child in an above-the-elbow cast for 3 weeks for an occult elbow fracture will not cause him or her any significant limitations once the cast is removed. The cast serves to help control the child's pain as well as prevent a probable nondisplaced fracture from becoming displaced. No further workup is necessary because the results will most likely not change the management of the injury.

References

1. Landin LA. Fracture patterns in children: analysis of 8,682 fractures with special reference to incidence, etiology and secular changes in a Swedish urban population 1950-1979. *Acta Orthop Scand Suppl.* 1983;202:1.
2. Goswami GK. The fat pad sign. *Radiology.* 2002;222:419-420.
3. Skaggs DL, Mirzayan R. The posterior fat pad sign in association with occult fractures of the elbow in children. *J Bone Joint Surg Am.* 1999;81:1429-1433m.
4. Major NM, Crawford ST. Elbow effusions in trauma in adults and children, is there an occult fracture? *AJR Am J Roentgenol.* 2002;178(2):413-418.

How Do You Perform a Fasciotomy of the Forearm?

Rachel S. Rohde, MD

The first key to performing a successful forearm fasciotomy is recognizing that a patient has a compartment syndrome. Although some rely on compartment pressure measurements to make this diagnosis, I base my decision on clinical suspicion. Several symptoms and signs can be associated with compartment syndrome, the most reliable being pain out of proportion to injury and a tense arm. Paresthesias, weakness, and pain with passive motion of the fingers also are common. In obtunded patients or in the setting of equivocal examination, compartment pressures can be measured.[1] A pressure within 30 mmHg of diastolic can be used as an indication for compartment release. When you make the diagnosis, do the procedure emergently; 68% of patients undergoing fasciotomy within 12 hours of onset had functional extremities compared to only 8% treated after 12 hours.[2] Keep in mind that not all compartment syndromes are due to trauma; anything that causes decreased compartment volume (obtunded patient lying on limb, burns, tight dressings, excessive traction) or increased compartment swelling (coagulopathy, reperfusion injury, seizures, tetany, burns, cold, snakebites, excessive exercise, venous obstruction, renal disease, capillary leak syndrome, infection, injection or extravasation, rhabdomyolysis, Duchenne's muscular dystrophy) can result in compartment syndrome.[3]

Technique

The patient is placed in a supine position and the operative extremity is placed on a hand table. I apply a nonsterile tourniquet to the upper arm but only inflate it if a vascular injury is identified and bleeding needs to be controlled. Prep and drape the arm as far proximally as possible so that you can extend the incision to the upper arm if necessary.

Figure 7-1. Volar incision that allows decompression of all relevant volar structures.

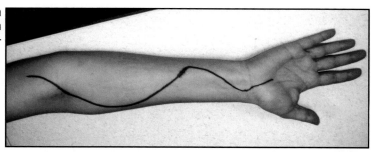

Figure 7-2. Volar incision that allows decompression of all relevant volar structures.

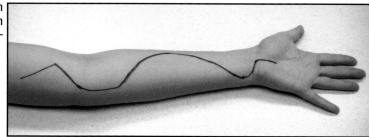

The anatomic compartments in the forearm include the superficial volar, deep volar (flexor digitorum profundus, flexor pollicus longus, and pronator quadratus), dorsal compartment, and the mobile wad (brachioradialis and extensor carpi radialis brevis and longus). You need to decompress all of these to ensure a good outcome.

Several different incisions have been described. Essentially, the goals of your incision are: 1) to allow complete decompression of all compartments and exploration of neurovascular structures, 2) to avoid injury to the palmar cutaneous branch of the median nerve, 3) to minimize risk of contracture at creases, and 4) to diminish exposure of nerves and vessels within open wounds. Figures 7-1 and 7-2 depict two commonly used incisions (note that each extends distal to the carpal tunnel and proximal to the lacertus fibrosis in the antecubital fossa).

I make the entire skin and subcutaneous tissue incision. I release the carpal tunnel with a fresh blade, incising the palmar aponeurosis and the transverse carpal ligament. This provides an excellent view of the median nerve distally.

I then return to the antecubital fossa area, where I divide the lacertus fibrosis, a fascial continuation of the biceps tendon; here I can determine brachial artery flow. Continuing distally, I release the superficial flexor compartment in its entirety. I retract the flexor carpi ulnaris medially with the neurovascular bundle, examining integrity of the nerve and vessel; the flexor digitorum superficialis and median nerve are retracted laterally to expose the deep compartment. The deep volar compartment is very vulnerable to ischemic injury and must be released! Following release of the superficial and deep volar compartments and mobilization of each muscle, I examine the median nerve for compression at two additional sites—the proximal pronator teres and the proximal flexor digitorum superficialis.

After complete release of these compartments using a volar incision, the dorsal compartment rarely needs to be decompressed, unlike in the lower extremity. Often, release of the volar compartments decompresses the dorsal compartment as well. However, if

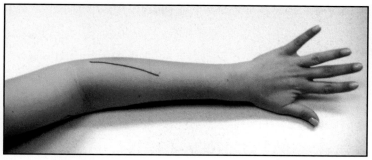

Figure 7-3. Dorsal incision that allows decompression of dorsal extensor compartment and mobile wad.

tension remains dorsally, I make a straight longitudinal incision extending from 2 cm lateral and 2 cm distal to the lateral epicondyle, approximately 10 cm long toward the middle of the wrist (Figure 7-3). Dorsal fascial incisions decompress the extensor compartment and mobile wad.

In some cases, hand fasciotomies are required. If there is considerable edema or pressure in the hand or if revascularization of the upper extremity has been performed, the hand should be addressed. Make a longitudinal incision over the 2nd and 4th metacarpals; a small hemostat can be inserted through these incisions and spread to release the dorsal and volar interosseous and adductor compartments between all metacarpals. Separate thenar and hypothenar incisions can be made along the glabrous borders of the hand and a hemostat can be used to decompress the thenar and hypothenar compartments. These incisions should be left open until edema has resolved.

I assess muscle viability by both color (pink vs dusky) and contractility to electrocautery stimulation. Debriding all necrotic tissue prevents infection and late contracture. If there is a question about the viability, I plan for return to OR in 2 or 3 days for repeat assessment, irrigation, and debridement.

Injuries to neurovascular structures should be repaired. Fascia should be left open. I always close the carpal tunnel incision. Additional skin should not be forced to close at the initial operation. I always cover nerves, vessels, and tendons (flexor retinaculum area) if possible. For temporary "closure" of swollen skin wounds, I usually use crisscrossed rubber bands with staples over a nonadherent mesh. Others leave skin edges free and apply bulky dressings. I have used vacuum dressings on lower extremities but prefer not to in the forearm, especially if there is any risk of nerve dessication.

I splint these patients postoperatively for comfort but minimize circumferential dressings and rely on frequent serial neurovascular examinations. Hand therapy is usually started on postoperative day 1 for tendon gliding and range of motion exercises to prevent stiffness and contracture.

Debridements are performed every 2 to 3 days until either the wound can be closed without tension or covered with split thickness skin graft.

References

1. Gelberman RH, Garfin SR, Hergenroeder PT, et al. Compartment syndrome of the forearm: diagnosis and treatment. *Clin Orthop.* 1981;161:252-261.

2. Sheridan GW, Matsen FA. Fasciotomy in the treatment of the acute compartment syndrome. *J Bone Joint Surg.* 1976;58:112-117.
3. Gulgonen A. Compartment syndrome. In: Green DP, Hotchkiss RN, Pederson WC, Wolfe SW, eds. *Operative Hand Surgery.* 5th ed. New York, NY: Churchill Livingstone; 2005:1985-2005.

CAST, EXTERNAL FIXATOR, OR OPEN REDUCTION AND INTERNAL FIXATION FOR A NONARTICULAR DISTAL RADIUS FRACTURE IN A 60-YEAR-OLD FEMALE?

John J. Fernandez, MD, FAAOS

In selecting treatment for a distal radius fracture, I consider four principal variables: associated soft-tissue injury, fracture reduction, fracture stability, and patient demands. These variables can be assessed through patient history, physical exam, and initial radiographs. In most cases, a treatment decision can and should be made prior to attempts at fracture reduction.

Soft-Tissue Injury

A thorough assessment of the soft tissues is integral in selecting treatment and should not be overlooked. The soft tissues comprise the envelope surrounding the distal radius: the tendons, nerves, and skin and subcutaneous tissue.

Swelling of the soft tissues may preclude treatment with a cast secondary to difficulty in achieving or maintaining a reduction. This may also impact the timing of surgical treatment. Even if closed-treatment is initiated, the soft tissues must be reassessed, as swelling can worsen after initial fracture reduction. Swelling can predispose complications of stiffness, carpal tunnel syndrome, and complex regional pain syndrome.

If there are signs and symptoms of nerve injury or entrapment such as carpal tunnel syndrome, a surgical release may be indicated and this would preclude cast treatment.

Fracture Reduction

The success of treatment is predicated on the quality and stability of the reduction. If the fracture cannot be properly reduced, then treatment will fail regardless of the stability of the fracture or the chosen form of fixation. While some patients may tolerate residual deformity, there is a relationship between deformity and function. Depending on the patient's expectations, even small amounts of residual deformity can lead to an unacceptable cosmetic appearance or functional outcome.

Fracture alignment is assessed primarily with plain radiographs. There are four suggested radiographic views: PA and lateral in neutral rotation, and 45-degree pronated and supinated oblique views. If the initial radiographs are unacceptable, it is important to repeat the studies as needed.

There are five radiographic measurements used in assessing fracture alignment: radial inclination, palmar tilt, radial length, radial shift, and articular congruity (Figures 8-1A through 8-1D). There have been many clinical and biomechanical studies examining the effects of deformity on outcome.[1-3] Although there is no consensus as to which parameter of deformity most closely correlates with outcome, there are guidelines that can be used in assessing the adequacy of a reduction (Table 8-1).

If fracture alignment is not acceptable, a closed-reduction is attempted. Initial closed treatment can be pursued if the reduction is successful and the soft tissue allow (Figures 8-2A and 8-2B). Follow-up examinations are repeated every few days or every week for the first 3 to 4 weeks. Surgical reduction and fixation is necessary if the closed-reduction fails initially or in subsequent follow-up.

Fracture Stability

The ability to maintain an acceptable reduction is proportional to the stability of the fracture. Fracture stability is multifactorial, but primarily based on energy of injury and quality of bone.

Energy of injury is proportionally dissipated into the bone and soft tissues. High-energy mechanisms, such as motor vehicle collisions, tend to create unstable fracture patterns. Low-energy mechanisms can also result in unstable fractures if bone quality is poor or the energy is focused on the wrist.

Fracture stability can be assessed from initial radiographs even prior to attempts at reduction. There have been studies attempting to quantify instability based on several factors.[4,5] Ultimately, the assessment should be a qualitative one based on clinical judgment. I evaluate a combination of factors pooled from these studies to help guide my decision (Table 8-2). If the fracture displays these characteristics, I deem the fracture unstable and recommend surgical fixation (Figures 8-3A through 8-3C).

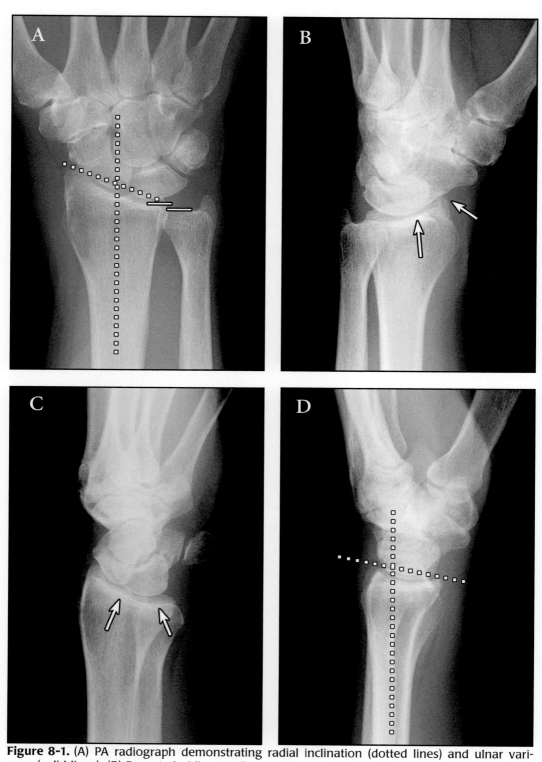

Figure 8-1. (A) PA radiograph demonstrating radial inclination (dotted lines) and ulnar variance (solid lines). (B) Pronated oblique radiograph imaging radial styloid and articular congruency. (C) Supinated oblique radiograph imaging volar-ulnar fragment and articular congruency. (D) Lateral radiograph demonstrating volar inclination (dotted lines).

Table 8-1
Predictors of Fracture Instability

- Age over 60 years
- Dorsal metaphyseal comminution
- Articular involvement
- Dorsal angulation greater than 20 degrees
- Loss in radial height
- Translation of volar cortex
- Associated ulna fracture
- Associated carpal injury
- Associated soft-tissue injury

Figure 8-2. (A) PA and lateral pre-reduction radiographs demonstrating comminution, loss in radial inclination, loss in radial height, and dorsal angulation. (B) PA and lateral postreduction radiographs demonstrating acceptable correction in alignment.

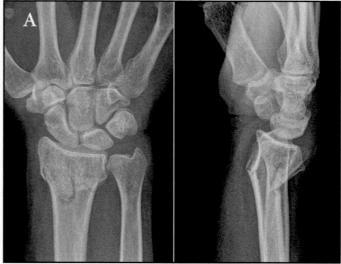

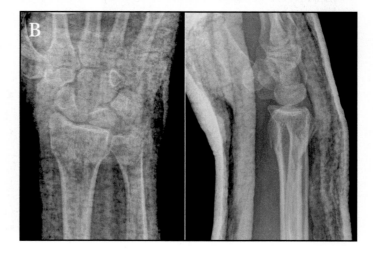

Table 8-2

Adequacy of Reduction

- Radial inclination greater than 10 degrees
- Ulnar variance less than 4 mm positive
- Palmar tilt less than 15 degrees dorsal or 20 degrees volar
- Articular congruity less than 2 mm gap or step-off

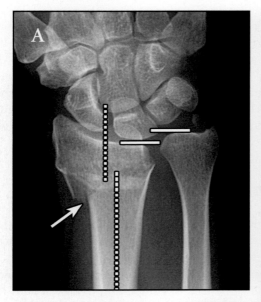

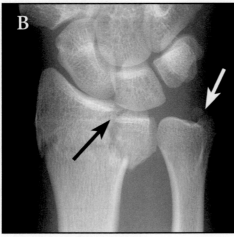

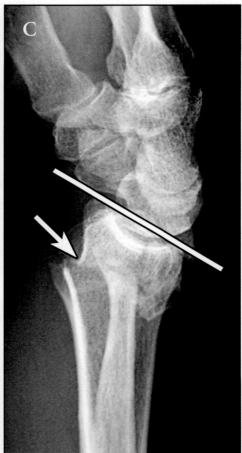

Figure 8-3. (A) PA radiograph demonstrating instability; loss in radial height (solid lines), communition (arrow), and radial translation (dotted lines). (B) PA radiograph demonstrating instability; ulna styloid fracture (white arrow) and articular involvement (black arrow). (C) Lateral radiograph demonstrating instability; dorsal collapse and angulation (solid line) and dorsal translation (arrow).

Patient Demands

In selecting treatment, perhaps the most important consideration is the patient's demands. Patient "demands" refer not only to the functional demands placed on the patient but also the demands the patient makes of the surgeon, ie, expectations. Even if there is a good functional and radiographic outcome, if the patient's expectations have not been met, the outcome could be considered a failure.

Account for the patient's independence, ie, does he or she live and shop alone? There is a correlation between increasing age and decreasing functional demands, but there are exceptions. Is this 60-year-old patient more like an 80-year-old or a 40-year-old? There may be concomitant medical conditions such as heart and lung disease, stroke, dementia, or arthritis that may have left the patient with few functional needs. Deformity may be well-tolerated in low-demand individuals and treatment should be modified accordingly.

Social factors such as time off of work, limitations during recovery, and speed of recovery may also be important to the patient. All options including their risks and benefits should be presented and the patient should become an active participant in deciding treatment.

Treatment Options

The treatment options must be viewed within the context of the surgeon applying the treatment. Because all surgeons will have different skill-sets and levels of experience, they must judge for themselves their own effectiveness in applying various treatments.

The literature is clear that surgical treatment is superior to cast treatment for displaced, unstable fractures. Until recently, there has been a lack of compelling evidence demonstrating a significant difference in outcomes between external fixation and internal fixation, specifically dorsal fixation. There are higher rates of infection, hardware failure, and nerve problems with external fixation, and higher rates of tendon complication and early hardware removal with internal fixation.

With the advent of volar fixed-angle plating, complications previously encountered with dorsal plating have been significantly diminished. There is now increasing evidence supporting superior outcomes with volar plating over other forms of treatment.[6-9]

Conclusion

Cast, external fixator, or open reduction and internal fixation (ORIF)? Any of these treatment options could be effectively utilized in this case. Cast treatment could be selected for the patient with the reducible, stable fracture, or if the patient could tolerate deformity. In the irreducible or unstable fracture, surgical fixation would be applied with the choice of fixation determined by the surgeon's preference and level of experience.

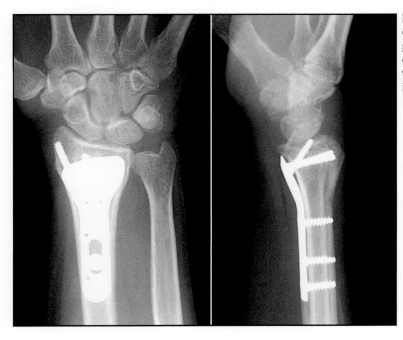

Figure 8-4. PA and lateral postoperative radiographs demonstrating correction in alignment with stable volar locking-plate fixation.

My preference is surgical fixation for all but the most stable or minimally displaced of fractures, even in some lower-demand patients. I find that most distal radius fractures in this age group are relatively unstable, even extra-articular fracture patterns. My choice of fixation is a volar fixed-angle plating system in all but the most severely of comminuted and displaced fractures (Figure 8-4). Even in cases of acceptable initial reduction, I present the patient with the option of surgical fixation including its risks and benefits. I find that volar fixed-angle plating allows for a more consistent and reproducible recovery with added patient comfort.

References

1. Pogue DJ, Viegas SF, Patterson RM, et al. Effects of distal radius fracture malunion of wrist joint mechanics. *J Hand Surg Am.* 1990;15:721-727.
2. Park MJ, Cooney WP III, Hahn ME, Looi KP, An KN. The effects of dorsally angulated distal radius fractures on carpal kinematics. *J Hand Surg Am.* 2002;27:223-232.
3. Kihara H, Palmer AK, Werner FW, Short WH, Fortino MD. The effect of dorsally angulated distal radius fractures on distal radioulnar joint congruency and forearm rotation. *J Hand Surg Am.* 1996;21:40-47.
4. Lafontaine M, Hardy D, Delince P. Stability assessment of disal radial fractures. *Injury.* 1989;20:208-10.
5. Mackenney PJ, McQueen MM, Elton R. Prediction of instability in distal radius fractures. *J Bone Joint Surg Am.* 2006;88:1944-1951.
6. Kreder HJ, Agel J, McKee MD, Schemitsch EH, Stephen D, Hanel DP. A randomized, controlled trial of distal radius fractures with metaphyseal displacement but without joint incongruity: closed reduction and casting versus closed reduction, spanning external fixation, and optional percutaneous K-wires. *J Orthop Trauma.* 2006;20:115-121.
7. Wright TW, Horodyski M, Smith DW. Functional outcome of unstable distal radius fractures: ORIF with a volar fixed-angle tine plate versus external fixation. *J Hand Surg Am.* 2005;30:289-299.
8. Orbay JL, Fernandez DL. Volar fixation for dorsally displaced fractures of the distal radius: a preliminary report. *J Hand Surg Am.* 2002;27:205-215.
9. Orbay JL, Fernandez DL. Volar fixed-angle plate fixation for unstable distal radius fractures in the elderly patient. *J Hand Surg Am.* 2004;29:96-102.

WHEN DO YOU REPLACE THE RADIAL HEAD?

Mark S. Cohen, MD
Robert W. Wysocki, MD

Radial head fractures account for approximately one-third of fractures about the elbow and are frequently associated with other elbow injuries including ulnohumeral dislocation; coronoid fracture, medial, and lateral collateral ligament injury; and interosseous membrane disruption. Optimal treatment requires an accurate understanding of the fracture pattern and proper diagnosis of associated elbow injuries.

The most common classification of radial head fractures is that of Mason. Type I fractures have less than 2 mm of intra-articular displacement and no mechanical block to motion. They can be treated with a short period of immobilization followed by aggressive range of motion. Type II fractures have either greater than 2 mm of intra-articular displacement or a mechanical block to motion. These are best treated with open reduction and internal fixation (ORIF). Type III fractures are complete articular fractures with comminution. A Type IV fracture, which has more recently been added, has an associated ulnohumeral dislocation. Unfortunately, this classification scheme has been shown to have poor reliability and reproducibility due to the difficulties in imaging a three-dimensional object with uniplanar radiographs. As such, when in doubt, advanced imaging with computed tomography can be useful in selected cases.

The most controversy in radial head fracture management lies in how to treat the comminuted fractures and those associated with instability of the elbow (fracture dislocations). The incidence of fracture comminution and elbow instability increases as the energy imparted increases. Thus, Type III and IV fractures are commonly seen in association. In series specifically addressing comminuted radial head fractures, concomitant elbow instability is present in 50% to 80% of cases. In this setting, radial head excision is contraindicated. With the presence of any indicators of instability (elbow dislocation, a significant coronoid fracture, axial or varus-valgus laxity), the radial head's role in load-bearing and as a secondary stabilizer to valgus load must be restored to maintain elbow and forearm stability. Thus, when treating fracture dislocations, the two options available are ORIF versus replacement arthroplasty.

Radial head excision may still be an option in the treatment of comminuted radial head fracture in an otherwise stable elbow. Biomechanical studies have reported increased valgus laxity as well as external rotation of the ulna in relation to the humerus after radial head excision with intact ligaments.[1] The clinical implications of these findings are not clear. Although such patients treated with excision have not been shown to have a significant risk for clinically relevant instability, they will often have weakness in grip and forearm loading. If instability at the time of injury is missed and the patient is treated with radial head excision, the consequences can be severe with several studies reporting uniformly poor results with early arthrosis and valgus instability rates of over 75%.[2,3] The patient and treating physician must be cognizant of these risks before proceeding with excision. As such, there is a recent trend toward radial head replacement when fractures are deemed irreparable.

ORIF of comminuted radial head fractures can be tedious and requires meticulous implant placement so as to provide stable fixation but not impinge on forearm rotation. Ring et al[4] have helped clarify which of these two options to choose based on the number of fragments. They reported no early failures and only one nonunion with uniformly good forearm range of motion after ORIF in 12 patients who had two to three articular fragments. Conversely, 13 of 14 patients with more than 3 articular fragments had an unsatisfactory result. Thus, the surgeon planning on treating a comminuted radial head fracture with ORIF should have arthroplasty implants available and be prepared to convert to radial head replacement in the face of an increasing number of articular fragments or an unexpected degree of comminution (Figure 9-1).

Metallic radial head arthroplasty has been shown in the laboratory to be capable of restoring normal elbow kinematics and stability both with intact ligaments as well as with ruptured ligaments after repair.[1] The earlier generation silicone implants were unable to restore valgus stability and thus are no longer used. Early clinical series have demonstrated good results with metallic implants both with and without concomitant elbow instability.[5-7] However, the implant wear properties and the long-term effect of the metal bearing on the articular surface of the capitellum are unknown and if improperly sized implants are used ("overstuffing"), maltracking, impingement, and early arthrosis can occur. There continues to be controversy in implant design including free-floating versus press-fit stems and monobloc versus bipolar components.

Mason Type IV radial head fractures seen in association with elbow dislocation are common, as radial head fracture occurs in 10% of elbow dislocations. These injuries require treatment not only of the radial head but also of the other stabilizing structures of the elbow that are injured.[8] Surgical treatment of the radial head with ORIF or arthroplasty is indicated if the fracture is displaced or if greater than 30% to 40% of the joint surface is involved. Once the radial head is repaired or replaced, the lateral soft tissues need to be meticulously repaired. Most commonly, part or all of the lateral ligament and extensor tendon origins tear off of their humeral origin.[9] Reconstitution of elbow stability requires repair of this sleeve back to the humerus. In more unstable cases, medial soft-tissue repair may also be required.

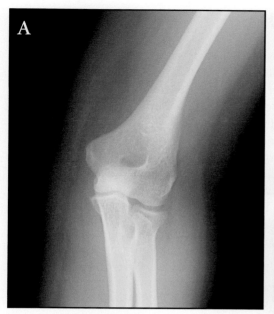

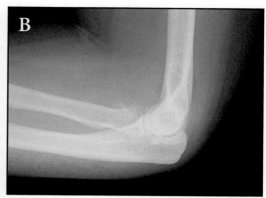

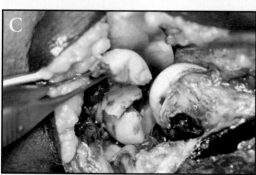

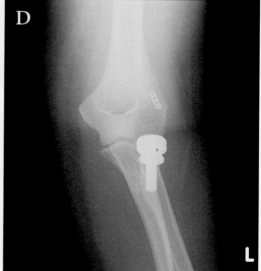

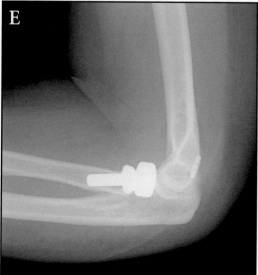

Figure 9-1. Anteroposterior (A) and lateral (B) radiographs demonstrating what appears to be a minimally displaced radial head fracture. Intraoperative photograph (C) showing substantial comminution at the time of surgery, for which arthroplasty (D and E) was eventually required.

Conclusion

A comminuted radial head fracture is most commonly a surgical injury. Without associated elbow instability, excision is still a viable option but carries known risks and over time may become obsolete as the results of arthroplasty become better defined. ORIF should be attempted for all comminuted fractures with two to three articular fragments that can be anatomically reconstructed. In this scenario, ORIF has shown excellent clinical results and avoids the aforementioned uncertainty still associated with arthroplasty.[4] For the unreconstructible radial head fracture with associated elbow instability, radial head arthroplasty is required and attention must be paid to the other injured stabilizing structures. For irreparable cases without instability, arthroplasty is an option with promising early results. As longer follow-up becomes available and the risks and implant designs become better understood, radial head replacement may become the standard of care for unreconstructible radial head fractures.

References

1. Beingessner DM, Dunning CE, Gordon KD, Johnson JA, King GJ. The effect of radial head excision and arthroplasty onelbow kinematics and stability. *J Bone Joint Surg Am.* 2004;86-A(8):1730-1739.
2. Broberg MA, Morrey BF. Results of delayed excision of the radial head after fracture. *J Bone Joint Surg Am.* 1986;68(5):669-674.
3. Josefsson PO, Gentz CF, Johnell O, Wendeberg B. Dislocations of the elbow and intraarticular fractures. *Clin Orthop Relat Res.* 1989;(246):126-130.
4. Ring D, Quintero J, Jupiter JB. Open reduction and internal fixation of fractures of the radial head. *J Bone Joint Surg Am.* 2002;84-A(10):1811-1815.
5. Grewal R, MacDermid JC, Faber KJ, Drosdowech DS, King GJ. Comminuted radial head fractures treated with a modular metallic radial head arthroplasty. Study of outcomes. *J Bone Joint Surg Am.* 2006;88(10):2192-2200.
6. Moro JK, Werier J, MacDermid JC, Patterson SD, King GJ. Arthroplasty with a metal radial head for unreconstructible fractures of the radial head. *J Bone Joint Surg Am.* 2001;83-A(8):1201-1211.
7. Pugh DM, Wild LM, Schemitsch EH,King GJ, McKee MD. Standard surgical protocol to treat elbow dislocations with radial head and coronoid fractures. *J Bone Joint Surg Am.* 2004;86-A(6):1122-1130.
8. Cohen MS, Hastings H II. Acute elbow dislocation: evaluation and management. *J Am Acad Orthop Surg.* 1998;(1):15-23.
9. McKee MD, Pugh DM, Wild LM, Schemitsch EH, King GJ. Standard surgical protocol to treat elbow dislocations with radial head coronoid fractures. Surgical technique. *J Bone Joint Surg Am.* 2005;87(suppl 1, pt 1):22-32.

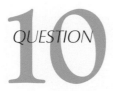

THERE IS A PATIENT IN THE ER WITH A FEMUR FRACTURE AND HUMERAL SHAFT FRACTURE. SHOULD I FIX THE HUMERUS WITH A NAIL OR A PLATE?

Timothy Bhattacharyya, MD

In a polytrauma patient presenting with a femur fracture and humeral shaft fracture, there is a relative indication to operate on the humerus to allow early mobilization. Fixation of the humeral shaft fracture will allow the patient early shoulder and elbow range of motion, and will allow early weight bearing on the extremity. This is extremely helpful, especially in the case of an ipsilateral humerus fracture and femur fracture.

Plate fixation is the best option. Randomized prospective studies have demonstrated that plate fixation of humeral shaft fractures result in lower reoperation rates, and earlier time to union.[1,2]

Intramedullary (IM) nailing of the humerus, while teleologically attractive, has not proven to be as reliable as nailing of tibial or femur fractures. Insertion of the humeral nail invariably involves injury to the rotator cuff, which results in shoulder pain in >50% of cases.[3] The structure of the humeral shaft does not provide a good isthmus, and rigid fixation is not possible. Locking the nail proximally and distally has a high rate of nerve injury. If IM nailing is chosen, antegrade or retrograde insertion is possible, depending on the location of the fracture. Antegrade nailing is done through a split created in the rotator cuff. Retrograde nailing avoids the rotator cuff, but is more technically challenging and is associated with residual elbow pain in some cases. In either case, the distal locking must be done through a small open approach to minimize nerve injury near the elbow.

I begin by performing the femoral nail (Figure 10-1). After that is completed, if the patient is stable, I proceed to open reduction and internal fixation (ORIF) of the humeral shaft. Usually, this is done on a hand table, which can be attached to the fracture table or radiolucent table. The table is turned 90 degrees. The standard Henry approach to the humeral shaft provides extensile exposure. A limited contact dynamic compression plate

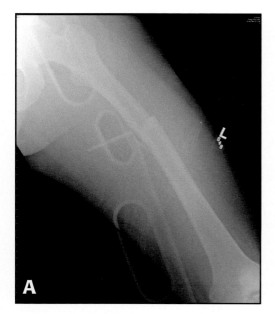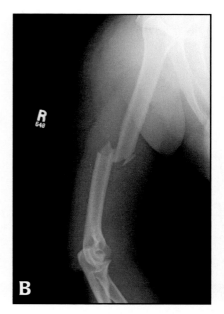

Figure 10-1A, B. A 41-year-old admitted after MVA with (A) femoral shaft and (B) humeral shaft fracture.

of 4.5 mm or its equivalent should be used. Large fragment screws provide excellent fixation, and the 4.5-mm plate size is necessary to allow early weight bearing. If the patient is large, a staggered configuration can be used, otherwise a 4.5 narrow plate functions as well. Six cortices of fixation should be obtained proximal and distal to the fracture. For transverse fractures, it is necessary to prebend the plate so that placement of screws in compression does not cause gaping of the side opposite the plate (Figure 10-2).

I reserve locking plate fixation for elderly patients (>70 years old) when poor quality bone is anticipated or when I am unable to get six cortices of fixation. With locking plates, I begin by obtaining reduction, securing with one conventional screw on each side of the fracture to bring the plate down to the bone and generate compression across the fracture site, then fill the remaining holes with locking screws.

The patient should be counseled preoperatively that a radial nerve palsy is possible. I generally do not visualize the radial nerve routinely from the anterior approach. If the patient has a radial nerve palsy preoperatively, I do not explore the radial nerve. The only exception to this rule is in the case of open fractures, where there is a higher rate of radial nerve laceration and exploration is beneficial.

If a 4.5-mm plate is used and good fixation obtained, I do not use any postoperative splinting and allow the patient to do shoulder and elbow range of motion as tolerated. They can weight bear as tolerated on the upper extremity.

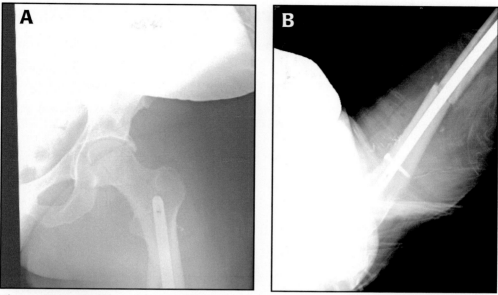

Figure 10-2. AP (A) and lateral (B) radiographs showing femur treated with a retrograde nail.

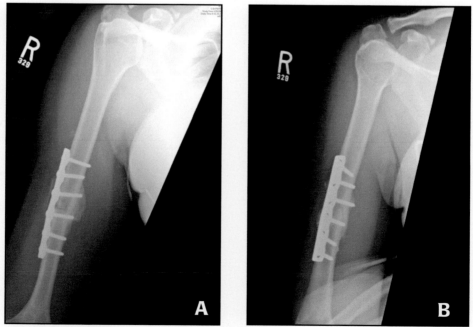

Figure 10-3. AP (A) and lateral (B) radiographs showing the humerus treated with ORIF.

References

1. Chapman JR, Henley MB, Agel J, Benca PJ. Randomized prospective study of humeral shaft fracture fixation: intramedullary nails versus plates. *J Orthop Trauma*. 2000;14:162-166.
2. McCormack RG, Brien D, Buckley RE, McKee MD, Powell J, Schemitsch EH. Fixation of fractures of the shaft of the humerus by dynamic compression plate or intramedullary nail. A prospective, randomised trial. *J Bone Joint Surg Br*. 2000;82(3):336-339.
3. Robinson CM, Bell KM, Court-Brown CM, McQueen MM. Locked nailing of humeral shaft fractures. Experience in Edinburgh over a two-year period. *J Bone Joint Surg Br*. 1992;74(4):558-562.

I HAVE A 30-YEAR-OLD PATIENT WHO HAD A POSTEROLATERAL DISLOCATION OF THE ELBOW. HOW WOULD YOU TREAT HIM?

Michael J. Medvecky, MD

The patient presenting with an acute posterolateral elbow dislocation typically sustains the injury from a fall onto an outstretched hand. An axial compressive force is applied onto the outstretched hand and as the body internal rotates on the fixed hand, external rotation and valgus forces are applied to the elbow. Due to the compressive forces, associated fractures can occur such as radial head and neck, capitellum, or coronoid.

Elbow dislocations can be classified into simple or complex—simple being purely ligamentous injuries (Figure 11-1) and complex being dislocations associated with periarticular fractures. O'Driscoll et al[1,2] have reviewed the theoretical pathoanatomy associated with ligamentous injury from dislocation, which can be thought of as a progressive soft-tissue injury in three stages. The injury is initiated laterally with tearing of the ulnar part of the lateral collateral ligament resulting in posterolateral rotatory subluxation (stage 1). As rotatory subluxation progresses, the coronoid can become perched onto the trochlea (stage 2). Progressive ligamentous injury is propagated medially as the dislocation ensues. The posterior part of the medial collateral ligament (MCL) tears, potentially leaving the anterior band of the MCL intact, which can become a pivot point for rotation (stage 3A). Progressive injury can occur to the anterior band of the MCL (stage 3B).

It is important to carefully assess for associated fractures in the radiographic analysis of these injuries—radial head and neck fractures, medial or lateral epicondyle fractures, and coronoid fractures are the most common. Additional fractures away from the elbow can occur as well, such as distal radius and ulnar styloid fractures, and hand and shoulder fractures. Associated soft-tissue injuries can also occur and careful neurologic examination should be documented pre- and postreduction.

Closed reduction is obtained under conscious sedation or general anesthetic. With the patient in the supine position, the forearm is supinated, shoulder is forward flexed, axial traction is applied to the forearm in order to clear the coronoid from the trochlea,

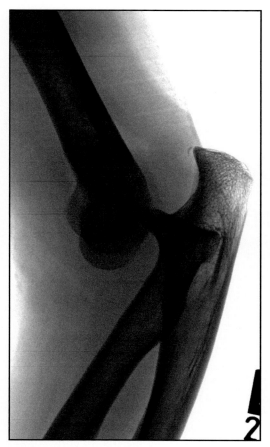

Figure 11-1. Lateral x-rays of the elbow demonstrating the posterolateral dislocation of the radius and ulna, without fracture.

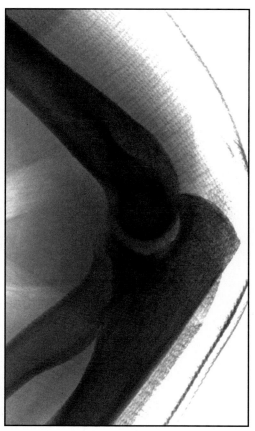

Figure 11-2. Lateral x-ray demonstrating reduction of the posterior elbow dislocation.

and the thumb of your opposite hand can be used to guide the olecranon process distally over the trochlea. The elbow is then examined for varus and valgus stability looking for competence of the anterior band at the MCL. Varus and valgus testing is done at multiple degrees of flexion starting at full extension up to about 60 degrees of flexion. The elbow is then assessed for stability in flexion and extension. The patient should have full flexion unless limited by soft-tissue swelling. The assessment of stability in extension is important information that should be documented postreduction, as it guides the rehabilitation plan.

After assessment of stability, the patient is placed into a padded posterior splint with the hand in pronation (Figure 11-2). Neurovascular examination is documented postreduction and assessment for neurovascular compromise should be done. If the elbow was stable to full extension postreduction, the patient can begin early range of motion. Those with instability in extension should be immobilized longer (approximately 2 weeks) or a hinged elbow brace with extension block mechanism can be placed. The patient is encouraged to begin early range of motion of the hand with isometrics of the flexors of the elbow and wrist. This increases the resting muscle tone and promotes compression through the elbow joint, conferring added stability and lessening subluxation. Patients with instability with extension are usually those with complete circumferential ligamentous injury including the anterior band of the MCL and should have protected range of motion with the hinged brace for up to 6 weeks.

Due to the results of elbow stability after nonoperative treatment of an acute simple elbow dislocation, acute operative ligamentous repair is rarely indicated.[3] It may be considered, however, if global instability is such that it does not permit early active protected motion in a brace. This is a more typical pattern with associated fractures and less common with a simple dislocation.

Postreduction follow-up is very important and the patient should be seen in the office a few days postinjury to assess for spontaneous redislocation that can occur even in a splint or cast.

Due to the ligamentous injury, postinjury scarring is likely to occur with some degree of associated elbow stiffness and variable degrees of extension greater than flexion loss. The patient immobilized longer than 3 weeks is likely to develop motion problems.[4] All patients should be alerted to expect some degree of extension loss.[5,6]

References

1. O'Driscoll SW, Bell DF, Morrey BF. Posterolateral rotatory instability of the elbow. *J Bone Joint Surg Am*. 1991; 73(3):440-446.
2. O'Driscoll SW, Morrey BF, Korinek S, et al. Elbow subluxation and dislocation. A spectrum of instability. *Clin Orthop Relat Res*. 1992;(280):186-197.
3. Osborne G, Cotterill P. Recurrent dislocation of the elbow. *J Bone Joint Surg Br*. 1966;48(2):340-346.
4. Garland DE, O'Hollaren RM. Fractures and dislocations about the elbow in the head-injured adult. *Clin Orthop Relat Res*. 1989;(168):38-41.
5. Mehlhoff TL, Noble PC, Bennett JB, et al. Simple dislocation of the elbow in the adult. Results after closed treatment. *J Bone Joint Surg Am*. 1988;70(2):244-249.
6. Morrey BF. *The Elbow and Its Disorders*. Philadelphia, PA: WB Saunders; 2000:933.

SECTION II

LOWER EXTREMITIES

My Patient Is 8 Years Old and Had a Salter-Harris III Fracture of the Distal Femur. How Long Should I Follow Him for Growth Abnormalities?

Andrea S. Kramer, MD

Physeal fractures are one of the unique aspects of pediatric orthopaedics. Injuries affecting the growth plate comprise 15% of all fractures in children. Injuries involving the epiphyseal plate can present special problems in management and diagnosis. Each physeal injury must be treated as a distinct entity, taking into account the patient's age, location of injury, type of injury, growth potential of affected area, degree of displacement, amount of initial trauma affecting the physis, and iatrogenic injury with late reduction. The Salter-Harris classification is useful for description and planning treatment, but it is the degree of displacement that will predict severity of complications and growth abnormalities.

Distal femoral physeal fractures often result from a hyperextension force. Up to 30% of patients can have growth disturbances and develop angular deformities. A greater force is required to produce an epiphyseal separation in the child than in the adolescent due to the thicker periosteum that provides greater stability. The chance of limb length discrepancy is greater in younger patients because this higher injury threshold results in more severe damage to the physis and there is a greater amount of growth remaining.

My approach to an 8-year-old with a Salter-Harris III fracture of the distal femur would first include understanding the morphology of the fracture, with multiple x-ray views and a CT scan using reconstructive images to best visualize intra-articular displacement.

One needs to carefully explain to parents the potential long-term complications involved with this type of injury, including growth arrest and angular deformities and the need for long-term follow-up. Nondisplaced fractures can be treated in a well-molded long-leg cast with the knee slightly flexed. I avoid extreme flexion to reduce the risk of neurovascular compromise. Displaced Salter-Harris III fractures require open, early,

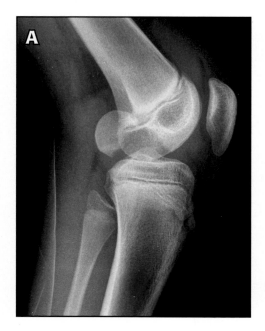

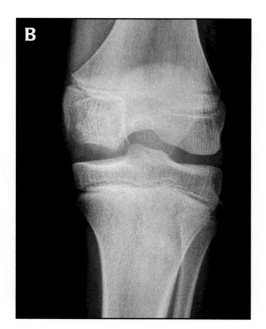

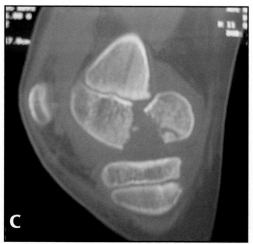

Figure 12-1. AP (A) and lateral (B) radiograph and sagittal CT scan (C) of a 12-year-old male with a Salter-Harris III fracture of the distal femur.

anatomic reduction under general anesthesia. Patients with late presentation or redisplacement should not undergo repeat reduction after 7 days to avoid iatrogenic physeal injury. In a nondisplaced Salter-Harris III fracture, percutaneous screw fixation is appropriate. Alternatively, when an anteromedial or anterolateral incision is made, provisional stabilization is obtained with k-wires and the screws are placed transversely across the epiphysis.

Angular deformities and limb length discrepancy are major concerns following a distal femur physeal fracture. Anatomic reduction is imperative without residual angulation. Explanation to parents must always include potential long-term implications, which include a 30% chance of limb length discrepancy of 2.0 cm or more, or varus or valgus deformity of 5 degrees or more.[1] It is crucial to emphasize that growth arrest is linked

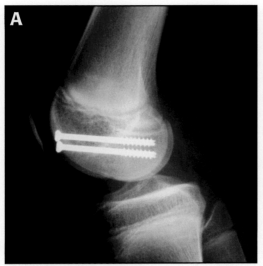 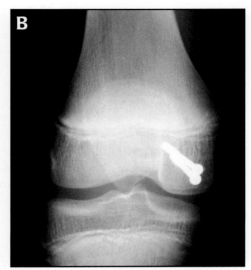

Figure 12-2. Postoperative lateral (A) and AP (B) radiograph of the distal femur showing anatomic reduction with countersunk lag screws.

to initial severity of the injury and amount of displacement, not the classification, and the likelihood of physeal disturbance is greater with significant (>50% of the width of the physis) initial displacement of the fracture.[2] Patients require close observation for development of a physeal bar and growth arrest. I obtain radiographs at 1 week, 6 weeks, 3 months, 6 months, and 1 year postop. If there is no evidence of physeal problems after the first 12 months, patients are then followed annually until skeletal maturity.

A complication unique to physeal injuries is growth disturbance producing angular deformity or shortening. Reconstructive procedures may be necessary for some patients, including physeal bar resection, contralateral epiphysiodesis, lengthening, or angular correction with stapling or osteotomy. Evaluation includes serial x-rays, including a standing mechanical axis or scanogram. Physeal injury may become noticeable as early as 6 months. Radiographs may show loss of normal physeal contours, loss of definition between epiphysis and metaphysis, sclerosis, or asymmetric Harris growth arrest lines. If x-rays are suspicious, I use magnetic resonance imaging (MRI) to assess bony bridging, evaluate residual physis, and map the injured physis. Alternatively, helical computed tomography (CT) scan is useful if available. Serial exams at 6, 12, 18, and 24 months will allow early detection of growth disturbances.

Growth arrests are considered to be complete or partial. Complete growth arrest in an 8-year-old will cause a significant limb length discrepancy, and therefore one must understand how to predict a future growth discrepancy. The distal femoral physis normally grows at a rate of 9 mm per year, the proximal tibia at 6 mm per year. It is generally agreed that a predicted discrepancy of <2 cm can be ignored, 2 to 5 cm are treated by epiphysiodesis of the opposite side, and if greater than 5 cm, a limb lengthening may be performed.

Angular deformity following distal femoral physeal injury is reported in approximately 24% of patients.[3] At age 8 years, more force is required to cause an epiphyseal separation than in an adolescent because the thicker periosteum provides greater stability, so there is a greater possibility of growth disturbances. Partial growth arrests or transphyseal bars can be difficult to treat. If the bar affects less than 30% of the total area of the physis, there is at least 2 years of growth remaining in the physis, and the deformity is less than 20 degrees, a bar resection may result in resumption of normal growth and gradual correction of the deformity. If angular deformity is greater than 20 degrees, corrective osteotomy may need to be performed, but my preference in an 8-year-old would be to proceed with a hemiepiphysiodesis using staples or plate to correct the angular deformity. It is less invasive than osteotomy, has a shorter recovery time, and allows remaining growth to help correct the deformity. Overall, several treatments are possible to treat growth disturbances.

References

1. Lombardo SJ, Harvey JP. Fractures of the distal femoral epiphyses. Factors influencing prognosis. A review of thirty-four cases. *J Bone Joint Surg.* 1977;59-A:742-751.
2. Riseborough EJ, Barrett IR, Shapiro F. Growth disturbances following distal femoral physeal fracture-separations. *J Bone Joint Surg.* 1983;65-A:885-893.
3. Beaty JH, Kumar A. Current concepts review: fractures about the knee in children. *J Bone Joint Surg Am.* 1994;76-A:1870-1880.

WHAT IS YOUR INITIAL EVALUATION OF PELVIC FRACTURES?

Andrew J. Furey, MSc, MD, FRCSC
Robert V. O'Toole, MD

High-energy pelvic ring disruptions are often associated with multiple injuries and may represent a potentially life-threatening insult.[1,2] As with any high-energy trauma patient, the initial assessment and hemodynamic stabilization of the patient should be directed by the Advance Trauma Life Support (ATLS) protocol.[3] Pelvic fractures typically require aggressive resuscitation. However, unlike most trauma patients, the orthopedic surgeon plays an important role in helping to determine the most likely source of bleeding for patients in shock and in helping to direct the initial management.

The first parameter to assess is the hemodynamic status of the patient. If the patient has a closed pelvic ring injury and is hemodynamically stable, there is no urgency in the acute management of the patient. You may review patient factors and complete imaging studies including anterior-posterior (AP) pelvis, inlet and outlet radiographs, and computed tomography (CT) scan before embarking on definitive treatment. Patients with pelvic ring injury require a particularly careful examination to rule out open fractures that may present through wounds in the rectum or vagina, as well as a detailed neurological examination and thorough secondary survey to find associated fractures and injuries. If indicated, operative fixation is typically performed within the first few days at our center. Vigilance is required with these patients, as hemodynamically stable patients can decompensate during their initial hospital course.

In contrast to the hemodynamically stable patient, the patient with hemodynamic instability despite adequate resuscitation requires the most prompt orthopedic evaluation and potential treatment. The first step is to evaluate the AP pelvis radiograph and determine if the pelvic volume is increased, as in a so-called "open book" pelvic fracture. This is an important distinction, as hemodynamically unstable patients with an increased pelvic volume (Figure 13-1) are at greater risk for life-threatening pelvic hemorrhage

Figure 13-1. AP pelvis radiograph demonstrating a pelvic ring injury with increased pelvic volume.

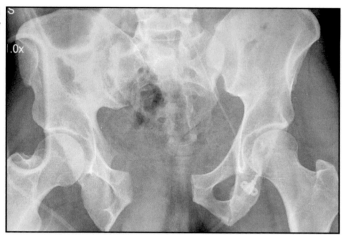

Figure 13-2. AP pelvis radiograph demonstrating a pelvic ring injury without an increased pelvic volume (same patient from Figure 13-1 after application of a binder).

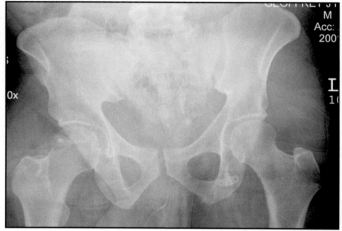

versus those with injuries that reduce the volume of the pelvis, regardless of the pelvic classification.

If the hemodynamically unstable patient has an increase in pelvic volume (Figure 13-1), then a closed reduction maneuver should be performed as quickly as possible using a compressive device. The compressive device will close the volume of the pelvis (Figure 13-2), help stabilize fracture fragments, and promote clot stabilization. The positive effects of such a device on a hemodynamically unstable patient are often dramatic; therefore, its application should be given the highest priority behind only the airway and breathing in these hemodynamically unstable patients. There are several compression devices available, including pelvic binders, bed sheets, external fixators, C-clamps, and MAST devices. We use pelvic binders in the acute setting, but a bed sheet is probably equally effective. If you are unsure if the pelvis volume is increased or you do not have a radiograph and only note pelvic injury by physical exam, we believe that it is appropriate to err on the side of placing a pelvic sheet when in doubt. The binder or sheet is centered at the greater trochanters and may be left in place for approximately 24 hours. Note that significant force is generated and frequent skin checks are essential to avoid skin breakdown. Holes can be cut in a binder for femoral lines or even for a laparotomy. Taping the knees together also can aid in the reduction.

Once the sheet is in place, a radiograph must be taken to ensure the volume of the pelvis has been reduced (Figure 13-2). If the pelvic volume has not been adequately reduced and the patient remains hemodynamically unstable, then the binder may be readjusted. If this fails, consider an emergent placement of an external fixator to assist in the reduction of the volume. This is a very rare situation and the emergency use of external fixation has essentially been completely replaced in our institution by binders.

Once the binder has been applied, and if the patient becomes and remains hemodynamically stable, the definitive fixation of the pelvic ring may proceed in a less emergent fashion. If, on the other hand, the patient remains unstable in a binder with radiographs confirming the adequate reduction of the pelvic volume, then angiography is the next appropriate step.

Indications for angiography in patients with pelvic injuries include continued hemodynamic instability despite reduction of pelvic volume in a binder and hemodynamic instability with a blush on CT. Angiography can be time-consuming, so you must be familiar with your own institution in terms of mobilizing the appropriate personnel in a timely fashion.

Finally, there is a subset of patients who are hemodynamically unstable and the volume of the pelvis is not increased, and in fact may be diminished. These patients do not typically benefit from a binder and the orthopedist can help alert the team to continue the search for other possible causes of continued hypotension. The exception to this rule is the geriatric patient, who due to calcified vessels may bleed significantly from seemingly innocuous fracture patterns. If there is no identifiable etiology of the hemodynamic instability, patients may benefit from angiography; however, as with any pelvic fracture, ensure that all other sources of blood loss and coagulopathy have been excluded and the resuscitation has been adequate.

Open pelvic ring injuries and associated injuries may affect the initial treatment. Open pelvic fractures carry a significant mortality rate and they must receive emergent irrigation, debridement, stabilization, and typically a diverting colostomy to facilitate wound care. Genitourinary injuries including urethral and bladder injuries are often associated with pelvic ring injuries and their treatment requires a combined approach with urology. The hemodynamically unstable pelvic fracture with intraperitoneal fluid is usually treated with emergent exploratory laparotomy, often in concert with orthopedics to place either temporary or definitive fixation.

The initial management of high-energy pelvic fractures requires a unique multidisciplinary approach, with the orthopedic surgeon intimately involved from the initial evaluation. One potential initial treatment algorithm is presented here (Figure 13-3), but the optimum treatment path is dependent on resources and expertise available at your institution.

References

1. Tile M, Helfet D, Kellam J. *Fractures of the Pelvis and Acetabulum*. 3rd ed. Philadelphia, PA: Lippincott Williams and Wilkins; 2003.

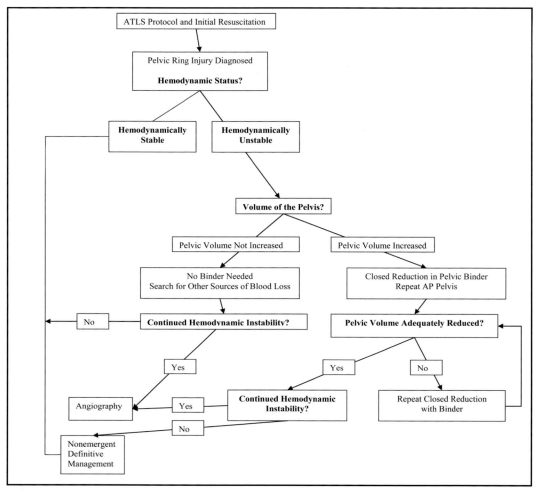

Figure 13-3. An algorithm for the initial management of a typical closed pelvic ring injury. The best algorithm for your institution depends on the expertise and resources available and other details of the patient's injuries.

2. Bucholz RW, Heckman JD. *Rockwood and Green's: Fractures in Adults*. 5th ed. Philadelphia, PA: Lippincott Williams and Wilkins; 2001.
3. American College of Surgeons. *Advanced Trauma Life Support Student Manual*. Chicago, IL: American College of Surgeons; 1997.

WHICH PELVIC FRACTURES ARE LIFE-THREATENING?

Andrew R. Burgess, MD

Orthopedic management of a trauma patient presenting with a pelvic fracture is maximized by appropriate resuscitation techniques based on the "ABCs" of resuscitation. Additional resuscitative measures can also be delivered to minimize the effects of associated pelvic hemorrhage.

Although exsanguination from an isolated pelvic injury is rarely singularly responsible for death, pelvic hemorrhage associated with other injuries is often a lethal combination. Therefore, while a high-risk pelvic fracture (grossly unstable, greatly displaced, unstable vital signs) needs immediate intervention (stabilization, angiography), so does a moderate-risk pelvic injury in a multiply injured patient. This clinical approach can be considered as minimizing the deleterious effects of the pelvic injury on the overall patient. In such a case, it is the orthopedist's task to take the effects of the pelvic injury "out of the equation," for example by rapid application of a pelvic binder to an unstable pelvis with an increased diameter as a trauma workup progresses.

Soon after the overall patient assessment and treatment of airway, breathing, and circulation has been performed, assessment of pelvic stability and injury mechanism should follow. This includes 1) manual and 2) radiographic assessment, and 3) a quick review of the circumstances of the injury. These three points are the most accurate determination of a life-threatening pelvic injury.

Assessment of Pelvic Injury

With the patient supine on a resuscitation litter permitting plain x-ray, the examiner will gently manipulate the pelvis via the anterior superior iliac spines toward and away from the midline. Detectable motion or significant pain should dramatically heighten

Figure 14-1. Inlet pelvis radiograph demonstrating a lateral compression type injury. Note the internal rotation of the right hemipelvis.

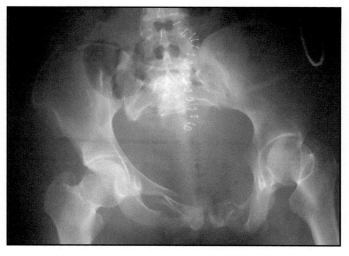

the suspicion of a significant pelvic injury. It is important to note the starting position of the pelvis prior to manipulation and the direction of instability. Radiographic evaluation must include anterior-posterior (AP), inlet and outlet radiographs, and computed tomography (CT) scan. Although significant displacement of fractures indicates severe injury, lesser degrees of displacement do no preclude severe injury, as the pelvis can recoil to a seemingly stable position. In general, significant anterior fracture displacement, significant deformity, and posterior ring fracture or dislocation suggests significant pelvic injury.

Lateral Compression Injuries

If physical exam reveals instability toward the midline, this signifies internal rotation or lateral compression instability. This is usually secondary to an injury caused by lateral compression displacing the hemipelvis toward the midline, such as a T-bone motor vehicle crash or a pedestrian struck from the side. A plain x-ray or CT scan indicating laterally applied compression, an available history of the event provided by EMTs or other witnesses, along with the physical exam, give the clinician quick insight into the personality of the pelvic fracture. In the case of a lateral compression fracture (Figure 14-1), anterior (transverse pubic rami) and posterior (often sacral) fractures, perhaps associated rib and pulmonary injury, solid viscous abdominal injury, genital-urinary injury and, in severe circumstances, aortic dissection or high cervical spine injury often present as a pattern.[1,2] If this type of patient is hypotensive or demonstrates signs of ongoing decompensation, stabilization of the pelvic ring will likely not add significant benefit. I believe the pelvic injury in such patients is not the source of significant hemorrhage and stabilization techniques often recreate the pathologic position of lateral compression injuries; that is, increasing the deformity and decreasing in pelvic diameter. Field or ER application of binders or sheets does not seem to cause additional harm, even though they exacerbate the original internal rotation deformity.

Elderly patients, unlike the majority of patients with lateral compression injuries, may have significant hemorrhage from injuries to the arterial branches of the posterior

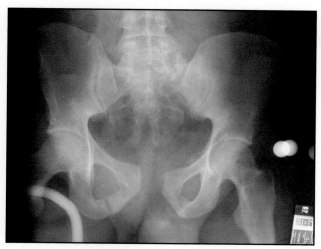

Figure 14-2. AP pelvis radiograph demonstrating an AP compression type injury. Note the widened symphysis and left sacral fracture. This injury can be associated with significant pelvic hemorrhage.

division of the internal iliac artery. This may be secondary to the "stiff sidewalls" of these vessels, causing them to transect when a shearing, lateral compression force is applied.

Anterior-Posterior Compression Injury

In a second example, the physical exam may seem similar, but the patient's pelvis is unstable or displaced in an external, open book position—an AP compression injury (Figure 14-2). Moving the ASIS toward the midline reduces the diameter of the true pelvis toward the normal anatomic position. These patients often present with hypotension and other physiologic and anatomic signs of severe injury. Radiographs show a widening of the pubic symphysis or rami fractures, and a displaced sacral fracture or SI joint dislocation posteriorly. Immediate stabilization of the patient's pelvis should be performed with a sheet or binder. This temporarily takes the pelvic injury out of the equation while the remainder of the resuscitation and workup proceeds. As the workup proceeds, other sources of hemodynamic instability may be discovered. Quickly applied pelvic ring stabilization is often followed by interventional angiography. Stabilization, such as application of a sheet or pelvic binder, should be performed prior to angiography or CT, as continued unabated pelvic venous bleeding responds well to decreasing the diameter of the true pelvis, as well as providing stabilization of the primary clot.

Identification of the life-threatening pelvic injury with 100% certainty is not possible. The above clinical approach combining physiologic, anatomic, and radiographic evaluation is the most useful emergent approach and will maximize survival, yielding a patient ready for more definitive treatment of the pelvic injury when appropriate.

References

1. Dalal SA, Burgess AR, Siegel JH, et al. Pelvic fracture in multiple trauma: classification by mechanism is key to pattern of organ injury, resuscitative requirements, and outcome. *J Trauma*. 1989;Jul29(7):981-1000.
2. Young JW, Burgess AR, Brumback R, Poka A. Pelvic fractures: value of plain radiography in early assessment and management. *Radiology*. 1986;160:445-451.

HOW DO YOU DECIDE WHICH PELVIC FRACTURES NEED SURGERY?

Scott A. Adams, MD, FRCS
Steven J. Morgan, MD, FACS

Pelvic ring disruptions represent a spectrum of injury, extending from the stable insufficiency fracture in the osteoporotic elderly patient, to the significantly displaced unstable fracture in the young patient involved in a motor vehicle accident (Figure 15-1).

The treatment of all patients with pelvic ring injuries begins with resuscitation. A standard trauma workup is required to identify concurrent injuries and evaluate the hemodynamic status. The indications and timing of fixation for pelvic fractures falls into two categories: emergent stabilization and definitive stabilization with internal fixation. In some instances, mechanically unstable pelvis injuries experiencing hemodynamic instability require acute intervention in the form of pelvic external fixation or a binder during the initial resuscitation. In the definitive phase, planned surgery strives to restore anatomic alignment or prevent the development of deformity. This surgical phase utilizes a combination of external or internal fixation to achieve these goals.

The vast majority of pelvic ring injuries occur in the elderly. The majority of these injuries represent the uncomplicated pubic rami fracture and account for about three-quarters of all pelvic ring injuries. These can be treated with analgesia, weight bearing as tolerated, and assessment of social circumstance. In young patients, however, the epidemiology of the pelvic fracture is different. These fractures are likely to be mechanically unstable, requiring definitive fixation, and often present with signs of hemodynamic instability that requires acute surgical intervention.

The current classification systems for pelvic injury attempt to predict the mechanical stability of the fracture pattern. Evaluation of pelvic stability in combination with assessment of patient comorbidities and associated injuries helps guide the treating physician in the decision-making process. The Young and Burgess[1] and Tile[2] classification systems define pelvic injuries according to the likely mechanism of injury and mechanical

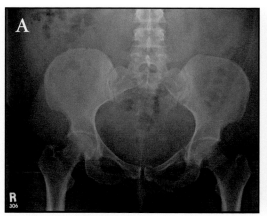 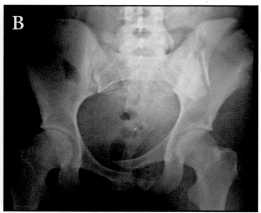

Figure 15-1. (A) Rami fracture (LC I) radiograph; (B) LC III injury radiograph.

stability. In the Young and Burgess system, injuries are divided into anteroposterior compression injuries (APC), lateral compression injuries (LC), vertical shear injuries (VS), and combined mechanism injuries (CM). APC injuries are typically due to a direct blow to the front or back of the pelvis, while LC injures are thought to be due to an insult from the side, such as a T-bone motor vehicle accident. APC and LC patterns are divided into three subtypes (I, II, and III) with increasing pelvic instability. VS and CM injuries usually occur in falls from heights, and these tend to be highly unstable both hemodynamically and mechanically. In addition to determining pelvic instability, this system can predict likely associated injuries and resuscitation requirements—APC, VS, and CM injuries are coupled with pelvic hemorrhage while LC and VS patterns are associated with abdominal viscera and head injuries. Tile's system[2] aids in predicting outcomes and treatment options—Type A fractures are stable, Type B rotationally unstable, and Type C vertically unstable.

During the initial trauma workup of the hemodynamically unstable patient with a pelvic injury, physiological parameters, physical examination of the pelvis, imaging studies, and history of the mechanism of injury will direct any resuscitative measures. AP, inlet and outlet radiographs, and computed tomography (CT) scan should be evaluated in cases of a displaced pelvic fracture to determine the need for surgical stabilization. Opinions and treatment algorithms vary between institutions and are often related to the resources and surgical experience available. However, emergent pelvic stabilization often with external fixation and angiography is part of all protocols used to treat the unstable patient with an unstable pelvis.

Identification of mechanically unstable pelvic ring injuries requiring fixation is reliant on accurate classification (Table 15-1). Using the Young and Burgess[1] classification, APC and LC Type I injuries can be managed nonoperatively with analgesia, weight bearing as tolerated, and close follow-up. In APC injuries where there is more than 2.5 cm of widening of the pubic symphysis, there is usually posterior injury, typically an open SI joint, and we feel operative management is indicated. Similarly, LC II and III injuries both have posterior involvement, the Type III being bilateral, and both require operative

Table 15-1

Young and Burgess Classification of Pelvic Ring Injuries and Treatment[1]

Classification	Subtype	Features	Treatment
APC	APC Type I	Diastasis < 2.5 cm	Usually managed nonoperatively.
	APC Type II	Diastasis > 2.5 cm Anterior SI ligament injury, posterior elements intact	Emergent stabilization for hemodynamic instability, utilizing pelvic binders or external fixators. Definitive fixation using external fixation or symphyseal plating anteriorly.
	APC Type III	Complete dissociation of the hemipelvis	Emergent stabilization for hemodynamic instability, utilizing pelvic binders or external fixators. Definitive fixation using external fixation or symphyseal plating anteriorly and a combination of closed reduction and percutaneous screw placement or open reduction and fixation for posterior injury.
LC	LC Type I	Anterior ring injury with a stable posterior lesion	Usually managed nonoperatively.
	LC Type II	Anterior ring injury with an unstable fracture dislocation of the sacrum or iliac wing	Emergent stabilization for hemodynamic instability, utilizing pelvic binders or external fixators. Definitive fixation using external fixation or plating of the fracture anteriorly and a combination of closed reduction and percutaneous screw placement or open reduction and fixation for posterior injury.
	LC Type III	LC I or II on side of injury with the addition of and APC type injury on the contralateral side	Combination of treatment for the LC II lesion plus the contralateral open book injury.
VS	VS	Vertical displacement of the hemipelvis	Emergent stabilization for hemodynamic instability, utilizing pelvic binders or external fixators, may require traction acutely. Definitive open internal fixation usually required.
CM	CMI	Aspects of all the above	Treatment based on primary injury vector.

Figure 15-2. Postoperative LC III injury radiograph.

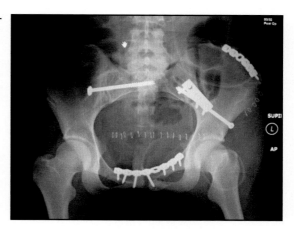

fixation (Figure 15-2). The VS and CM injuries often require stabilization emergently but also benefit from definitive operative management once hemodynamically stable. The Tile classification suggests nonoperative management for Type A, while B and C require surgical intervention.

Definitive fixation of mechanically unstable injuries takes place once the patient has responded to resuscitative measures, any associated injury has been stabilized, and the systemic inflammatory response to injury has normalized. Katsoulis and Giannoudis,[3] in a recent review on timing of pelvic fixation, suggest that fixation should take place after the fourth postinjury day to avoid further insult in the acute inflammatory phase and to allow the pelvic hematoma to consolidate, limiting further blood loss at the time of surgery. Techniques for definitive fixation are again guided by the fracture patterns and surgical experience. Debate continues on percutaneous versus open techniques, the use of external fixation for long-term management, and the order of fixation between the anterior or posterior ring when multiple sites of the pelvis are involved.

The timing of and indications for fixation of pelvic fractures continue to be perfected. The decision-making processes are helped by validated classification systems and local treatment algorithms. In general, the unstable pelvic fracture in the unstable patient is provisionally fixed emergently, while definitive fixation is ideally delayed until after day 4.

References

1. Young JW, Burgess AR, Brumback R, Poka A. Pelvic fractures: value of plain radiography in early assessment and management. *Radiology.* 1986;160:445-451.
2. Tile M. *Fractures of the Pelvis and Acetabulum.* Baltimore, MD: Williams and Wilkins; 2003.
3. Katsoulis E, Giannoudis, PV. Impact of timing of pelvic fixation on functional outcome. *Injury.* 2006;37(12):1113-1142.

I HAVE A 40-YEAR-OLD WITH AN ANTERIOR FRACTURE OF THE FEMORAL HEAD AND INCONGRUITY OF THE HIP JOINT. HOW WOULD YOU TREAT THIS?

Clifford Turen, MD
Andrew J. Furey, MSc, MD, FRCSC

Fractures of the femoral head represent a rare and challenging group of fractures. These difficult fractures have reportedly been associated with dislocations of the hip in 16% of cases.[1,2] These usually occur by direct impact of the femoral head on the edge of the acetabulum at the time of a dislocation. Depending on the exact position of the hip and the direction of the forces applied, a hip dislocation may be associated with an acetabular fracture, a femoral head fracture, or both.[3] The association between these injuries and a posterior hip dislocation often results in an anteromedial fracture fragment of the femoral head, which may or may not be attached to the ligamentum teres. The femoral head may also have an accompanying impaction injury.

There have been several classification schemes used to describe this unique set of injury patterns. The one most commonly used in the literature is the Pipkin classification, which is divided into four types: Type I fractures occur below the fovea and the ligamentum teres has been disrupted from the femoral head; Type II fractures occur above the fovea and the ligamentum teres remains attached to the fracture fragment; Type III fractures are femoral head fractures associated with femoral neck fractures; and Type IV fractures are femoral head fractures associated with an acetabular fracture. This classification, although not complete in its description, helps group fractures and provides a framework for surgeons to think about these injuries.

Once a femoral head fracture is suspected, we use a series of imaging modalities to help identify and describe the injury as well as assist in the direction of treatment. Initially, plain radiographs of the pelvis are used to identify the fracture, followed by a dedicated

Figure 16-1. AP radiograph of the pelvis demonstrating a left femoral head fracture with a small posterior wall fracture.

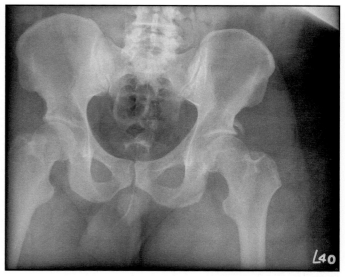

plain radiograph of the femoral neck and Judet radiographs to identify any associated femoral neck or acetabular fractures, respectively. If the hip remains dislocated and there is no femoral neck fracture, a gentle reduction is performed with the appropriate sedation and monitoring. If gentle closed reduction is not possible, one should proceed to open reduction emergently. If a closed reduction is achieved, the previously described images should be repeated. Following plain radiographic examination, we routinely investigate these fractures with computed tomography (CT) scans. We use the CT scan to examine the joint for congruency of the reduction, presence of intra-articular debris, presence of associated femoral neck or acetabular fractures, and to identify the exact location and amount of displacement of the femoral head fracture. Using these images, we formulate a treatment plan.

There are several treatment options a surgeon must consider when addressing these injuries. These include the following: nonoperative treatment, excision of the fragment, open reduction internal fixation (ORIF) through an anterior approach, or ORIF through a surgical hip dislocation.

Although historically popular, and well-described throughout the literature, non-operative treatment is currently rarely indicated for these fractures.[3] Since suprafoveal fractures involve the weight bearing articular surface, all suprafoveal fractures should be treated with anatomic ORIF. Infrafoveal fractures represent nonweight bearing cartilage, and one can accept less than anatomic position. However, these fractures will usually cause some degree of hip instability, alter hip mechanics, and are often associated with poor results if treated nonoperatively.[3] Therefore, we recommend surgical treatment of most infrafoveal fractures with either ORIF or excision of these fracture fragments, bearing in mind the possible instability from excision.

Once it has been decided that the patient requires surgical management, the next phase of the treatment plan involves formulating a plan for the surgical approach and the method of fixation. The main approaches employed for fixing these fractures are the Smith-Peterson approach and the surgical hip dislocation. We routinely use the Smith-Peterson approach and have not had significant issues with exposure; however, a surgical

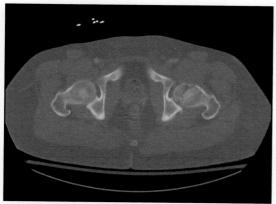

Figure 16-2. CT scan demonstrating the large femoral head fragment.

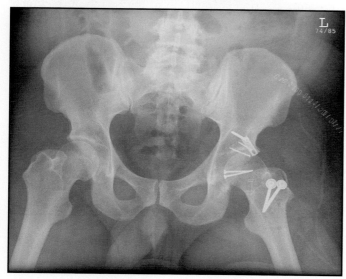

Figure 16-3. Postoperative AP pelvis radiograph demonstrating fixation of the two fractures through a posterior approach with a surgical dislocation. Note the two lag screws in the femoral head, the small plate on the acetabulum fracture, and the two large lag screws repairing the trochanter osteotomy done for the surgical dislocation.

dislocation offers a broader exposure to the entire femoral head and access to the posterior acetabulum. When performing a surgical dislocation, the surgeon should be intimately familiar with the anatomy of the blood supply to the femoral head.[3] When choosing the method of fixation, several options exist including countersunk screws, headless screws, and bioabsorbable fixation. We routinely use mini-fragment screws to minimize head size in addition to countersinking techniques for our fixation. Regardless of the fixation technique chosen, adequacy of reduction and appropriately buried hardware is critical.

In Pipkin I fractures, we will either perform an ORIF through a Smith-Peterson approach, or a surgical dislocation. The decision to excise or ORIF the fragment is based on the size of the fragment, its contribution to hip stability, and the degree of comminution present. If the fragment is necessary for hip stability, then ORIF is preferred; otherwise, excision may be considered. If there is excessive comminution present, then the fracture may not be reconstructable and excision may be the only option.

In Pipkin II fractures, we recommend ORIF through either a Smith-Peterson or a surgical dislocation to achieve absolute anatomic reduction and fixation with either headless screws or countersunk screws. These fractures occur in the weight bearing surface of the femoral head, requiring anatomic reduction and restoration of articular congruity.

Pipkin III fractures are very rare, with only a few reports in the literature. When assessing these fractures, the surgeon must also consider patient variables. It may be necessary to perform an ORIF of both the femoral neck and the femoral head, particularly in a young person. However, in an elderly individual, this associated injury pattern may best be treated with arthroplasty.

In Pipkin IV fractures, both injuries should be considered individually. The fractured acetabulum is usually a small fragment, and the decision to treat it should be based on the pattern of injury, hip stability, and quality of reduction. Likewise, the decision to treat the femoral head fracture should be based on its own characteristics. Caution should be applied in treating the femoral head nonoperatively or with excision in this situation, for it may render the hip unstable and require fixation of fractures of the acetabulum, which would otherwise be treated nonoperatively.

Postoperatively, we routinely limit weight bearing and institute posterior hip precautions depending on the fracture pattern and degree of stability assessed intraoperatively.

Conclusion

We recommend that most if not all fractures of the femoral head be treated surgically. There are several things one must consider in developing a treatment plan, including mechanism of injury, associated injuries, imaging modalities, surgical approaches, and types of fixation.

References

1. Epstein HC. Posterior fracture-dislocations of the hip: Long term follow-up. *J Bone Joint Surg Am.* 1974; 56:1103-1127.
2. Thompson VP, Epstein HC. Traumatic dislocation of the hip: a survey of two hundred and four cases covering a period of twenty-one years. *J Bone Joint Surg Am.* 1951;33:746-778.
3. Baumgaertner MR, Tornetta P. *Orthopedic Knowledge Update.* 3rd ed. Monmouth Junction, NJ: Rosemont; 2005.

17

I HAVE A 26-YEAR-OLD IN THE ER WITH A DISPLACED FEMORAL NECK FRACTURE. DO I NEED TO PERFORM AN OPEN REDUCTION AND CAPSULOTOMY?

Robert E. Blease, MD
Peter J. Nowotarski, MD

Unlike low-energy femoral neck fractures, which are seen frequently in the elderly and more sedentary population, similar fractures in younger patients generally indicate much higher energy injuries (Figure 17-1). Commonly, such injuries are the result of falls from a height or motor vehicle accidents. The converted femoral neck stress fracture, often seen with military recruits and athletes, is unassociated with a high-energy impact, but still seen in the young adult population. While the diagnosis and treatment protocol for hip fractures in the elderly is relatively straightforward, the same fracture in a young patient can present unique difficulties.

Although the displaced femoral neck fracture due to a high-energy injury will usually be quite evident, in the case of minimally displaced fractures such as those associated with femoral shaft fractures, the diagnosis is missed preoperatively up to 20% to 50% of the time. Despite being relatively infrequent, the disastrous consequences of a missed diagnosis and late displacement in this population has led to the proposal for a protocol to include dedicated internal rotation hip x-ray and dedicated fine cut computed tomography (CT) of the hip in patients with high-energy femoral shaft fractures.[1]

Once a diagnosis of displaced femoral neck fracture is made in a young patient, urgent treatment is indicated based on evidence suggesting a 2-fold (10.5% versus 20%) increase in the rate of osteonecrosis occurring in those patients treated more than 6 hours after time of injury as opposed to those treated prior to the 6-hour mark.[2] Although this evidence is based on a more elderly population in whom osteonecrosis is relatively easily treated with either femoral head resurfacing or hip arthroplasty, any resort to such measures in a younger patient can have devastating and life-altering consequences,

Figure 17-1. Displaced femoral neck fracture above ipsilateral shaft fracture (not pictured).

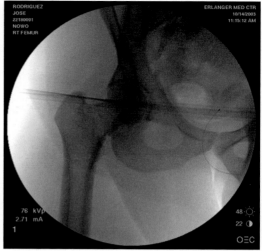

including multiple revision surgeries, complications, and degradation of quality of life. A more recent article challenges this 6-hour rule and sets the cutoff for worsening complications only if patients are surgically delayed by more than 48 hours.[3] If at all possible, we recommend the treatment of these injuries as soon as is practical with the goal of treatment less than 6 hours from the time of injury.[4]

Surgical treatment for these patients is generally performed under traction in either the lateral decubitus or in the supine position. The chosen position is a reflection of the surgeon's preference for either a Hardinge lateral, a Watson-Jones, or a Smith-Peterson approach, should open reduction be necessary. Our preferred approach is supine positioning with extraskeletal traction applied against a perineal post, and subsequent use of a Watson-Jones approach if required (Figure 17-2). Our reasoning for not performing a posterior approach is the increased risk to the critical vascular structures supplying the femoral head posteriorly. Regardless of the approach or position used, an anatomic reduction is required for these fractures in order to maximally restore hip kinematics, perfusion, and venous outflow.

If closed reduction can be obtained (generally through a combination of traction and internal rotation), then percutaneous fixation can be performed with either cannulated lag screws (6.5 mm in diameter or larger), a sliding hip screw construct with or without a derotational screw, or via a 130-degree blade plate. Biomechanical studies have demonstrated that a sliding hip screw with derotational screw is mechanically superior to the hip screw alone as well as to multiple lag screws or a blade plate. For a more stable, less vertical fracture pattern, we generally prefer to use three 7.3-mm lag screws with care taken to position the screws within the dense subchondral bone of the femoral head (Figure 17-3). For more unstable fractures to include those with a greater vertical sheer component, we prefer to use a sliding hip screw with a derotational screw (7.3-mm or 6.5-mm diameter). One additional option would be to use a three-screw construct following a transverse lag screw (ie, a Weber screw). Two recent, as yet unpublished, studies indicate that the new locking proximal femoral plates may prove to be mechanically superior to any of these constructs.

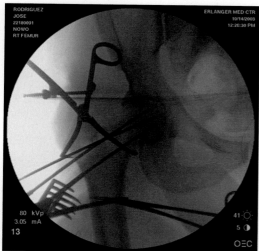

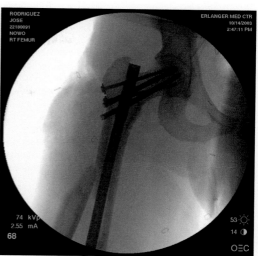

Figure 17-2. Intraoperative reduction via Watson-Jones approach, with initial passage of wires for cannulated screws.

Figure 17-3. Final construct—recon nail (for shaft fracture), with x2 cannulated screws to treat neck fracture.

The decision to perform a capsulotomy on a patient in whom a closed reduction has been obtained is not clearly indicated in the literature. Although multiple studies have recorded increased capsular pressure with subsequent hypoperfusion of the femoral head, most notably in displaced fractures, no definitive correlation has been established between these factors and the onset of osteonecrosis. If the hip capsule is thought to have remained intact, we prefer to perform a percutaneous capsulotomy in order to release intracapsular pressures and thus to re-establish normal blood flow to the femoral head. If an open reduction is necessary for adequate reduction, then capsulotomy is performed with the approach.

Complications most commonly consist of nonunion, avascular necrosis, and loss of fixation. One recent study indicated an overall rate of 19% of nonunion for all age groups, but notes increasing rates as age increases and higher rates for women in general. For the younger patient population, the risk is approximately 10%.[5] Treatment includes revision open reduction and internal fixation (ORIF), vascularized bone grafting, osteotomy, or arthroplasty. Loss of fixation is relatively less common and when it occurs is more likely related to initial poor implant placement. Treatment is dependent on the vascular status of the head, but is generally similar to that for nonunions. Avascular necrosis may be seen initially quite early, or as far out as 3 years or more after injury and treatment.

Conclusion

A displaced hip fracture in an otherwise healthy young patient constitutes a relative orthopedic emergency due to the high potential risk for AVN. We prefer rapid treatment of these injuries with an anatomic reduction performed closed or via anterior Watson-Jones approach. Capsulotomy is performed through the open reduction approach, or percutaneously if closed reduction is performed.

References

1. Tornetta P 3rd, Kain MS, Creevy WR. Diagnosis of femoral neck fractures in patients with a femoral shaft fracture. Improvement with a standard protocol. *J Bone Joint Surg Am.* 2007;89(1):39-43.
2. Szita J, Cserhati P, Bosch U, Manninger J, Bodzay T, Fekete K. Intracapsular femoral neck fractures: the importance of early reduction and stable osteosynthesis. *Injury.* 2002;33(suppl 3):C41-6.
3. Upadhyay A, Jain P, Mishra P, Maini L, Gautum VK, Dhaon BK. Delayed internal fixation of fractures of the neck of the femur in young adults. A prospective, randomised study comparing closed and open reduction. *J Bone Joint Surg Br.* 2004;86(7):1035-1040.
4. Shrader MW, Jacofsky DJ, Stans AA, Shaughnessy WJ, Haidukewych GJ. Femoral neck fractures in pediatric patients: 30 years experience at a level 1 trauma center. *Clin Orthop Relat Res.* 2007;454:169-173.
5. Parker MJ, Raghavan R, Gurusamy K. Incidence of fracture-healing complications after femoral neck fractures. *Clin Orthop Relat Res.* 2007;458:175-179.

18

WHAT IS YOUR CHOICE FOR A DISPLACED FEMORAL NECK FRACTURE IN A 65-YEAR-OLD: ORIF, HEMIARTHROPLASTY, OR TOTAL HIP ARTHROPLASTY?

Matthew L. Jimenez, MD

Displaced fractures of the femoral neck occur in elderly patients as a result of a low-energy fall. The mechanism of injury in younger patients is typically a higher-energy event such as a motor vehicle accident, motorcycle accident, or a fall from a height. Displaced femoral neck fractures in 65-year-old patients are caused by a variety of mechanisms due to this age groups' ever-increasing activity level and improvement in general health and well-being. Physiologic age and bone quality are more useful criteria than absolute chronologic age when determining a treatment strategy for displaced femoral neck fractures.

Diagnosis and Imaging

Unlike stress fractures and nondisplaced fractures of the femoral neck, displaced femoral neck fractures present with readily observable findings. Patients typically exhibit significant pain, shortening, and rotational deformity of the injured extremity. I prefer immediate traction in the emergency room using a soft boot and roughly 10 pounds of weight. This measure provides some pain relief, improves fracture alignment, and allows for a more useful radiograph, since an externally rotated limb at the time of x-ray does not show an appropriate view of the femoral neck. However, there is some evidence that keeping the leg in its "antalgic" position with minimal traction may decrease the intracapsular hip joint pressures, and theoretically have a positive impact on femoral head blood flow.

The initial radiographic evaluation should include an anterior-posterior (AP) and lateral radiograph of the injured hip. Ideally, the AP radiograph should be obtained with approximately 10 to 15 degrees of internal rotation to allow an orthogonal view of the femoral neck allowing for the proximal femoral anteversion. On the AP and cross-table lateral radiographs, I pay particular attention to the obliquity of the fracture line on the AP view, the presence or absence of posterior femoral neck comminution on the lateral radiograph, and the degree of hip joint degeneration. These radiographic characteristics influence treatment decisions.

Anatomy and Classification

The blood supply to the femoral head is at significant risk when a fracture of the femoral neck displaces. The femoral head derives its primary arterial blood supply from the lateral epiphyseal artery, which is the terminal branch of the medial femoral circumflex artery. The lateral epiphyseal artery is injured in displaced femoral neck fractures as it runs along the posterosuperior aspect of the femoral neck before terminating into several retinacular branches supplying the femoral head.

Multiple classification schemes exist for femoral neck fractures. I find the Garden (Figure 18-1) and Pauwels (Figure 18-2) classification systems most useful. The Garden classification for femoral neck fractures can be further simplified into undisplaced (Type I and II) and displaced (Type III and IV) injuries. The Pauwels classification divides femoral neck fractures by the obliquity of the fracture line relative to the horizontal. This system is useful when assessing the stability of a given fracture pattern, which determines type and position of fixation devices.

Surgical Treatment

I treat patients with displaced femoral neck fractures in their fifth and sixth decades of life with the same consideration as young patients with high-energy injuries. A healthy 65-year-old patient must not be grouped with the typical elderly low-energy osteoporotic fracture. Physiologic age is more important than chronologic age, and must be considered in light of the mechanism of injury, fracture pattern and displacement, associated injuries, and general medical comorbidities.

There is not complete agreement regarding the timing of surgery for displaced femoral neck fractures. I prefer to operate as soon as possible, taking into consideration the patient's general medical condition and appropriate medical clearance. Displaced femoral neck fractures adversely affect the blood flow to the femoral head; therefore, early anatomic reduction and stable internal fixation may improve femoral head blood flow. There is some evidence that early surgical intervention may decrease the risk of osteonecrosis of the femoral head.

ORIF

Open reduction and internal fixation (ORIF) is my primary treatment strategy for displaced fractures of the femoral neck in a healthy 65-year-old patient with good bone quality.

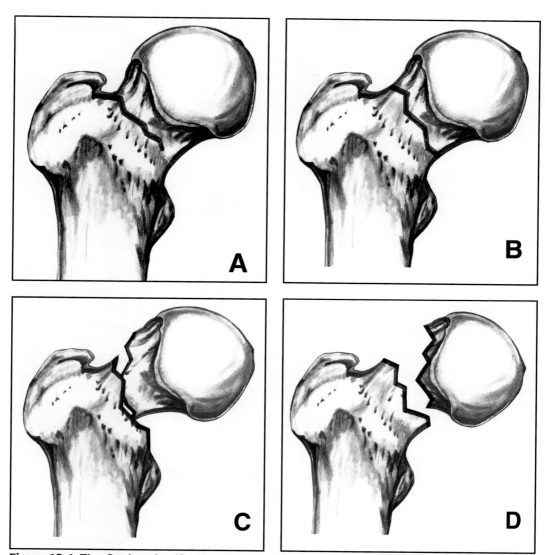

Figure 18-1. The Garden classification for femoral neck fractures groups injuries into Type I (A) incomplete impacted valgus, Type II (B) nondisplaced, Type III (C) incomplete displacement in varus, and Type IV (D) completely displaced fracture with no bone contact. For prognostic purposes, Type I and II can be grouped into nondisplaced and Type III and IV can be grouped into displaced, since fracture displacement carries greater risk for osteonecrosis of the femoral head. (Image art created by Matthew L. Jimenez, MD.)

An attempt at gentle closed reduction under fluoroscopic guidance is reasonable, although if closed reduction cannot be achieved, I move forward with open reduction. The surgical approach I find most useful is the modified Hardinge transgluteal lateral approach. The Watson-Jones anterolateral approach and the Smith-Peterson anterior approach offer alternative access to the femoral neck. A posterior approach to the hip should be avoided to maintain the important posterior blood supply of the femoral head.

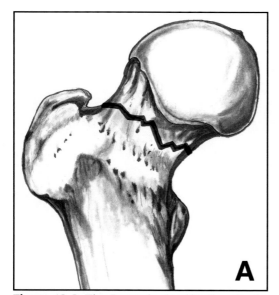
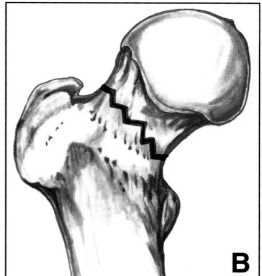
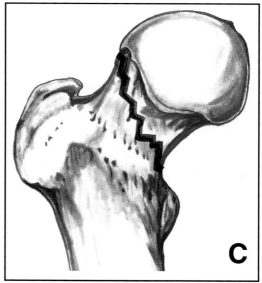

Figure 18-2. The Pauwels classification for femoral neck fractures divides injuries by the fracture angle relative to the horizontal. Type I (A) is relatively horizontal (<30°) and exhibit fairly stable compressive forces. Type II (B) is more oblique (30°-50°) and shear forces at the fracture site are increased. Type III (C) exhibits a steep fracture angle relative to the horizontal (>50°) and shear forces predominate. (Image art created by Matthew L. Jimenez, MD.)

Supine positioning with the leg prepped and draped free into the surgical field allows manual traction and rotation, which facilitates the fracture reduction. A radiolucent operating table and fluoroscopy are mandatory to confirm fracture reduction and implant position. Threaded half-pins are useful to "joy-stick" the femoral neck fragments into the appropriate alignment, and k-wires help my provisional fixation while confirming the reduction under direct visualization and intraoperative fluoroscopy. An anatomic reduction is the goal.

When choosing implant type, number, and configuration, I find the Pauwels classification helpful. For Pauwels Type I and II fractures, three cancellous lag screws provide optimal fixation. I attempt to place the screws as close as possible to the endosteal cortex of the femoral neck in an inverted triangle configuration to provide maximal resistance to rotation and shear. For Pauwels Type III fractures, and fractures with significant posterior femoral neck comminution, an additional cancellous screw placed superior in the femoral neck and head and parallel to the horizontal resists fracture displacement.

HEMIARTHROPLASTY VERSUS TOTAL HIP ARTHROPLASTY

Prosthetic replacement has a role in the treatment of displaced femoral neck fractures in the elderly patient with poor bone quality and comminution. I can achieve a more predictable result with prosthetic replacement in the elderly patient, compared to the higher failure rate observed with internal fixation, with the goal of pain relief and early mobilization.

Good to excellent results can be expected with either cemented or uncemented newer generation hemiarthroplasties. Considerable evidence comparing unipolar and bipolar bearings for elderly patients with displaced femoral neck fractures demonstrates no clear difference in morbidity, mortality, or functional outcome.

My indication for total hip arthroplasty for patients with displaced femoral neck fractures has been associated symptomatic ipsilateral hip joint arthritis. Recent evidence, however, has expanded the indications to include active elderly patients with displaced femoral neck fractures and otherwise normal hips because of more predictable pain relief and better function.

Bibliography

Bonnaire F, Schaefer DJ, Kuner EH. Hemarthrosis and hip joint pressure in femoral neck fractures. *Clin Orthop.* 1998;353:148-155.

Gautier E, Ganz K, Drugel N, Gill T, Ganz R. Anatomy of the medial femoral circumflex artery and its surgical implications. *J Bone Joint Surg Br.* 2000;82:679-683.

Swiontkowski MF. Intracapsular fractures of the hip. *J Bone Joint Surg Am.* 1994;76:129-138.

Szita J, Cserhati P, Bosch U, Manniger J, Bodzay T, Fekete K. Intracapsular femoral neck fractures: the importance of early reduction and stable osteosynthesis. *Injury.* 2002;33(suppl 3):C41-C46.

HOW WOULD YOU TREAT A VARUS FEMORAL NECK NONUNION IN A 50-YEAR-OLD?

Michael Garcia, MD
Michael D. Stover, MD

Varus femoral neck nonunion presents a therapeutic challenge, particularly in a growing middle-aged patient population. Intracapsular hip fractures are at risk for nonunion secondary to their biomechanical and biological environment. The femoral neck sees extremely high sheer forces along fracture lines that lie in line with the direction of force across the hip joint. Also, in intracapsular fractures, the lack of periosteum along with intervening synovial fluid does not allow for fracture healing through new bone (callus) formation. These fractures require anatomic reduction and compressive fixation to encourage primary bone healing, yet even in these ideal situations, fracture healing is not guaranteed.

Femoral neck fractures and their subsequent nonunions and risk of segmental osteonecrosis can lead to degeneration of both the femoral and acetabular joint surfaces. This adds another level of clinical complexity to this problem. Not only must the physician determine if the fracture can heal, but if healing is achieved, if the resultant joint surface will be functional for the patient.

In order to treat a nonunion of the femoral neck, the disadvantageous biomechanical environment must be changed. Typically, reorienting the fracture line in a more perpendicular position relative to the lines of force across the hip joint can provide this change. A valgus producing intertrochanteric osteotomy achieves the goal of improving the biomechanics of the fracture environment, while also having the ability to restore some proximal femoral anatomical relationships. The sheer forces seen by the fracture in its native position are converted to a more compressive force, thus providing a more advantageous environment for the fracture to heal. If the joint surface is preserved with adequate remaining motion, this is the option we typically prefer.

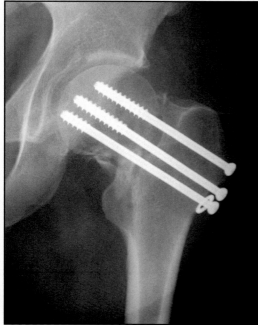

Figure 19-1. AP radiograph of a 53-year-old male's hip 9 months after fixation for a high-energy femoral neck fracture showing non-union and early hardware failure.

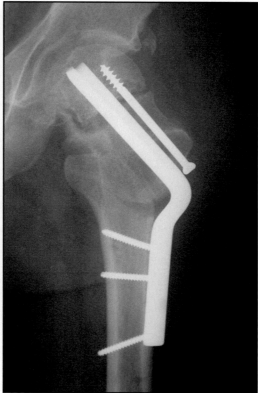

Figure 19-2. Immediate postoperative radiographs after valgus producing intertrochanteric osteotomy.

Most commonly at our institution, a fixed angle device such as a blade plate is used to fix the fracture and osteotomy site. This provides rigid internal fixation of the femoral neck and osteotomy site and also provides a reproducible amount of valgus correction allowing for preoperative planning and templating of the osteotomy. There are risks when performing this procedure, particularly the creation of a new fracture (the osteotomy) to fix a nonunited fracture, leaving open the possibility of the production of an iatrogenic nonunion. This is unlikely because the osteotomy is made in the metaphyseal, intertrochanteric region. Great care must be taken to adequately reduce and apply compression across the osteotomy site once the blade is in place. Marti et al[1] reported on 41 patients treated as above, showing 86% of the nonunions went on to heal with a 0% intertrochanteric nonunion rate. The functional outcomes were satisfactory as well with a mean Harris hip score of 91.[1] Other reports show similar results with union rates between 85% and 100% and improvements of the mean Harris hip score observed.[2,3] This is our procedure of choice, particularly in the young, active patient because it preserves the native hip joint (Figures 19-1 through 19-3).

Should the hip show signs of degeneration, we usually opt for reconstruction with total hip arthroplasty. Typically, this is performed through a direct anterior approach on a fracture table. This allows us to recreate the anatomic relationships of the patient's native

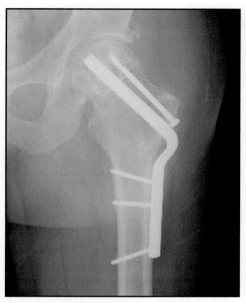

Figure 19-3. Seven-year follow-up radiographs showing complete consolidation of the fracture with excellent preservation of the joint space. Clinically, the patient has excellent hip function and is without complaints.

hip joint and enables us to unburden the active, young patient with the typical precautions inherent to other classically described surgical approaches.[4,5] Total hip arthroplasty takes away the two sources of pain for the patient, the nonunion site and the degenerated hip joint itself. It is a reproducible, reliable operation that has excellent long-term outcomes. There are several reports in the literature regarding outcomes of total hip arthroplasty using a multitude of techniques including cemented, hybrid, and all press-fit constructs. These show excellent long-term survivability of the prosthesis.[6-8] Increased acetabular liner wear, osteolysis, and reoperation rates are typically associated with the younger, more active patients. Alternative bearing surfaces beyond the typical metal on polyethylene constructs for use in the younger patient population have shown decreased osteolysis and aseptic loosening rates but long-term follow-up is not readily available. The long-term effects, both positive and negative, cannot be assessed.

In this clinical scenario, the patient is relatively young compared to the typical arthroplasty patient. Questions regarding the longevity of the prosthesis and subsequent revision surgery make arthroplasty a less than ideal choice. Therefore, if adequate bone material remains, we prefer a valgus producing osteotomy for this patient. Secondary surgery (ie, total hip arthroplasty) for failure of the osteotomy has been shown to be more difficult, but shows similar long-term outcomes to primary total hip arthroplasty.[10]

Conclusion

In conclusion, preservation of the native hip through osteotomy and fracture healing is our procedure of choice if adequate bone material is present. We use a blade plate to fix both the osteotomy and nonunion site, thus enabling us to provide rigid internal fixation with reproducible correction and high subsequent union rates. In cases of segmental osteonecrosis of the femoral head and significant bone destruction, we prefer total hip arthroplasty.

References

1. Marti RK, Schuller HM, Raaymakers ELFB. Intertrochanteric osteotomy for nonunion of the femoral neck. *J Bone Joint Surg Br.* 1989;71B:782-787.
2. Ballmer FT, Ballmer PM, Baumgartel F, et al. Pauwels osteotomy for nonunions of the femoral neck. *Orthop Clin North Am.* 1990;21:759-767.
3. Anglen JO. Intertrochanteric osteotomy for failed internal fixation of femoral neck fracture. *Clin Orthop.* 1997; 341:175-182.
4. Kennon RE, Keggi JM, Wetmore RS, et al. Total hip arthroplasty through a minimally invasive anterior surgical approach. *J Bone Joint Surg Am.* 2003;85A(suppl4):39-48.
5. Matta JM, Shahrdar C, Ferguson T. Single-incision anterior approach for total hip arthroplasty on an orthopaedic table. *Clin Orthop Relat Res.* 2005;441:115-24.
6. Engh CA, Culpepper WJ, Engh C. Long-term results of use of anatomic medullary locking prosthesis in total hip arthroplasty. *J Bone Joint Surg Am.* 1997;79:177-84.
7. Keener JD, Callaghan JJ, Goetz, DD, et al. Twenty-five-year results after Charnley total hip arthroplasty in patients less than fifty years old. *J Bone Joint Surg Am.* 2003;85:1066-1072.
8. Kim YH, Oh SH, Kim JS. Primary total hip arthroplasty with a second-generation cementless total hip prosthesis in patients younger than 50 years of age. *J Bone Joint Surg Am.* 2003;85:109-114.
9. Kim SY, Kyung HS, Ihn JC, et al. Cementless metasul metal on metal total hip arthroplasty in patients less than 50 years old. *J Bone Joint Surg Am.* 2004;86:2475-2481.
10. Haverkamp D, de Jong PT, Marti RK. Intertrochanteric osteotomies do not impair long-term outcome of subsequent cemented total hip arthroplasties. *Clin Orthop Relat Res.* 2006;444:154-60.

What Is Your Postoperative Management of Hip Fractures in the Elderly?

Daniel K. Laino, MD
Kenneth A. Egol, MD

As technical advances in fracture fixation have lead to faster, more successful recovery following hip fracture surgery, standardized clinical pathways have been developed to further improve outcomes. At our institution, we have found that initiation of a standardized clinical pathway for hip fracture management is associated with decreased acute hospital length of stay, in-hospital mortality, and 1-year mortality.[1]

Recovery Room

We routinely obtain a postoperative electrocardiogram (EKG) and general laboratory studies. Patients with a history of cardiopulmonary disease or those with postoperative EKG changes are placed on a rule-out myocardial infarction protocol that involves transfer to a monitored setting for observation by one of our medical intensivists. These high-risk patients receive serial EKGs and cardiac enzyme monitoring for 24 hours postoperatively.

It is widely accepted that hip fracture patients are at high risk for deep vein thrombosis (DVT). The American College of Chest Physicians currently recommends the following agents for prophylaxis against DVT in hip fracture surgery patients: fondiparinux, low molecular weight heparin (LMWH), low-dose unfractionated heparin (LDUH), or warfarin titrated to an international normalized ratio (INR) of 2:3.[2] Mechanical prophylaxis is recommended if anticoagulant-based prophylaxis is contraindicated because of increased risk of bleeding, or as an adjunct to anticoagulant-based prophylaxis.[2] Our typical protocol is to apply sequential compression devices (SCDs) in the recovery room immediately following surgery and begin chemoprophylaxis with fondiparinux 6 to 8 hours after surgery or enoxaparin 12 to 24 hours after surgery depending on attending preference. Patients receiving warfarin are given the first dose the night after surgery. It is recommended that hip fracture surgery patients receive extended prophylaxis for up to 28 to 35 days after surgery.[2]

For postoperative pain control, patient controlled analgesia (PCA) is utilized as long as patients can cooperate; otherwise, they are given injectable narcotics titrated to a level of comfort. Intravenous fluids are administered until the patient is able to tolerate a regular diet. Incentive spirometry and deep breathing exercises are initiated immediately following surgery in the recovery room.

Postoperative Day 1

On postoperative day 1, the urinary catheter and any suction drains are discontinued. Prophylactic antibiotics are continued for a total of 24 hours. There is no evidence to support continuation of prophylactic antibiotics beyond 24 hours even if the patient has retained drains or catheters.[3] IV fluids are discontinued if the patient is tolerating oral intake, and the patient is transitioned to oral pain medication. The patient's calves are examined daily for signs of tenderness or swelling and a duplex ultrasound is ordered if any abnormalities are present. We do not routinely screen for DVT in asymptomatic patients.[2]

Indications for blood transfusion following hip fracture surgery remain controversial.[4] We typically consider blood transfusion in patients with hemoglobin less than 9 mg/dL if the patient is symptomatic and has a lower threshold for transfusion, and in patients with preexisting cardiac disease. Perioperative allogenic blood transfusion has not been shown to significantly affect mortality, incidence of wound infection, or incidence of chest infection in hip fracture patients at 1-year follow-up.[5] All patients on warfarin receive daily PT/PTT monitoring and their warfarin dose is titrated to a therapeutic level (INR 2:3). Patients in the rule-out myocardial infarction protocol are transferred to a regular room as long as they are cleared for transfer by the medical team.

Physical therapy is initiated on the first postoperative day. Early ambulation is associated with accelerated functional recovery and shorter length of stay.[6] Patients who were treated with internal fixation have no restriction in hip range of motion. Those treated with prosthetic replacement are maintained on standard hip precautions. All patients are allowed weight bearing as tolerated.[7] On postoperative day 1, the patient is instructed on transfers and ambulation with assistive devices. We find that an overhead trapeze is essential because it assists with transfers in and out of bed. Goals are modified according to the patient's physical, psychological, and social situation, but early ambulation to includes stair climbing and strengthening is stressed.

Occupational therapy is also initiated on postoperative day 1. The occupational therapist assists the patient in regaining the ability to participate in activities of daily living (ADLs) such as cooking, bathing, dressing, and toileting. This is often done via the use of assistive devices. Long-handled reachers, shower benches, shoe horns, and stocking-aids assist patients in performing ADLs.

We find that most elderly patients will need a course of formal rehabilitation following operative fixation of a hip fracture. On postoperative day 1, a consultation is made to the rehabilitation service for evaluation for inpatient rehabilitation.

Postoperative Day 2 and Beyond

On postoperative day 2, suction drains and Foley catheter are discontinued if still present. Laxatives and stool softeners are given if constipation is an issue. By the third postoperative day, the patient is working with physical therapy twice daily and is out of bed to a chair as much as possible.

Delirium is a frequent complication of hip fracture in the elderly. Reduction of non-critical medication, active management of preexisting medical conditions, and treatment of postoperative complications (eg, urinary tract infections) are all important for prevention of delirium.[8] Regulation of bowel and bladder function, early mobilization, adequate nutritional intake, environmental stimulation (clocks, hearing aids, glasses, etc), pain control, and maximizing central nervous system oxygen delivery (maintaining adequate hematocrit, oxygen saturation, and blood pressure) are also measures that can help prevent and treat delirium.

We have several criteria for determining suitability for discharge from the hospital. First, patients should be hemodynamically stable, afebrile, and medically optimized. They should be tolerating a regular diet and pain should be well-controlled on oral medications. Finally, the patient should be "cleared" by the physical and occupational therapists, indicating a basic level of mobility, functioning, and ability to perform ADLs. Transfer to a rehabilitation or skilled nursing facility is often necessary, so appropriate referrals and arrangements will need to be made by the appropriate discharge planners.

References

1. Koval KJ, Chen AL, Aharonoff GB, Egol KA, Zuckerman JD. Clinical pathway for hip fractures in the elderly: The Hospital for Joint Diseases experience. *Clin Orthop Relat Res.* 2004;425:72-81.
2. Geerts WH, Pineo GF, Heit JA, Bergqvist D, Lassen MR, Colwell CW, Ray JG. Prevention of venous thromboembolism: the seventh ACCP conference on antithrombic and thrombolytic therapy. *Chest.* 2004;126:338-400.
3. Braztler DW, Houck PM. Antimicrobial prophylaxis for surgery: an advisory statement from the national surgical infection prevention project. *Clin Infect Dis.* 2004;38:1706-1715.
4. Carson JL, Terrin ML, Magaziner J, et al. Transfusion trigger trial for functional outcomes in cardiovascular patients undergoing surgical hip fracture repair (FOCUS). *Transfusion.* 2006;46:2192-206.
5. Johnston P, Wynn-Jones H, Chakravarty D, Boyle A, Parker MJ. Is perioperative blood transfusion a risk factor for mortality or infection after hip fracture? *J Orthop Trauma.* 2006;20:675-79.
6. Oldmeadow LB, Edwards ER, Kimmel LA, Kipen E, Robertson VJ, Bailey MJ. No rest for the wounded: early ambulation after hip surgery accelerates recovery. *ANZ J Surg.* 2006;76:607-611.
7. Koval KJ, Sala DA, Kummer FJ, Zuckerman JD. Post-operative weight-bearing after a fracture of the femoral neck or an intertrochanteric fracture. *J Bone Joint Surg Am.* 1998;80:352-356.
8. Robertson BD, Robertson TJ. Postoperative delirium after hip fracture. *J Bone Joint Surg Am.* 2006;88:2060-2068.

21

HOW WOULD YOU TREAT A FEMUR FRACTURE IN A 6-YEAR-OLD?

Pradeep Kodali, MD
John F. Sarwark, MD
Najeeb Khan, MD

A full evaluation using Advanced Trauma Life Support (ATLS) protocol in children and adolescents with a femur fracture should be used because they have a 35% to 40% incidence of associated injuries, including femoral neck fracture, hip dislocation, ligamentous instability of the knee, and visceral injuries.[1] Femoral shaft fractures represent approximately 2% of all pediatric fractures. The incidence is bimodal with peaks at ages 2 and 12 years.[2] Cortical thickness of the femur increases rapidly after 5 years of age, leading to decreased incidence of femur fractures in late childhood.

It is important to determine the mechanism of injury because a high-energy trauma is more likely to require surgical stabilization or prolonged immobilization. Child Protective Services should be called if nonaccidental injury is suspected. It is estimated that 42% of infants and 17% of patients younger than age 6 with femoral fractures have nonaccidental mechanisms.[2] A spiral fracture pattern does not necessarily indicate abuse.

In proximal fractures, the proximal fragment tends to flex, abduct, and externally rotate due to unopposed muscular forces. Any residual deformity is generally tolerated because of its proximity to the multidirectional hip joint and because the residual angulation is hidden in the thigh muscles. Supracondylar fractures assume an apex posterior angular deformity due to the pull of the gastrocnemius muscle. These fractures require precise alignment because coronal plane deformity, which is perpendicular to the sagittal axis of the joint, is not well-tolerated from both a functional and cosmetic standpoint.

The potential for remodeling is substantial in pediatric femur fractures until approximately age 12 in boys and age 10 in girls.[1] Up to 25 degrees of midshaft angulation in any plane can be expected to correct satisfactorily by remodeling in children younger than 13 years.[1]

High-energy fractures with severe displacement, comminution, or shortening greater than 3 cm require maintenance of length and alignment by spica cast, traction, external fixation, or internal fixation. Surgical stabilization with external or internal fixation techniques provides the advantage of early joint mobilization. Acceptable deformity ranges in this age group tend to be higher due to a greater potential for remodeling. Recommended guidelines are up to 15 degrees of varus or valgus, 20 degrees of anterior or posterior angulation, and up to 2 cm of shortening.[2] Surgical stabilization should be considered for fractures that exceed these guidelines and for unstable subtrochanteric fractures.

Children up to 10 years of age with low-energy femur fractures with less than 2 cm of shortening are good candidates for a spica cast. A spiral fracture pattern tends to do better with this treatment than a transverse. Under anesthesia, gentle axial compression under fluoroscopy should be done to verify that the fracture does not shorten more than 3 cm. Significant shortening of the fracture would make traction or surgical stabilization more appropriate than a spica cast. The optimal position of a spica cast is 90 degrees of hip flexion and 90 degrees of knee flexion with slight hip abduction. Follow-up visits at 1 and 2 weeks and then at 4 weeks are recommended to monitor alignment. The cast is discontinued when there is radiographic evidence of callus and absence of pain at the fracture site.

If the minimal canal diameter allows, our preference is to use flexible intramedullary nails in a 6-year-old (see Chapter 22 for insertion technique).

External fixation is a treatment option in any age group, and is generally recommended in polytrauma, open fractures, and very distal or proximal fracture femoral shaft fractures.

Skeletal traction is rarely required given the advances and availability of other techniques. However, if there is greater than 2 cm initial shortening, traction may be helpful to heal to appropriate length prior to spica cast application.[3] This may take 2 to 3 weeks.

Generally, fractures in children under 10 heal without any major complications. Patients in this age group do well with nonoperative treatment due to their potential for remodeling. Parents should be given both nonoperative and operative management options for treatment of these fractures.

References

1. Price CT, Flynn JM. Management of fractures. In: Morrissy RT, Weinstein SL, eds. *Lovell and Winter's Pediatric Orthopaedics.* Philadelphia, PA: Lippincott Williams & Wilkins; 2006.
2. Flynn JM, Schwend RM. Management of pediatric femoral shaft fractures. *J Am Acad Orthop Surg.* 2004;12: 347-359.
3. Anglen JO, Choi L. Treatment options in pediatric femoral shaft fractures. *J Orthop Trauma.* 2005;19(10):724-732.

HOW WOULD YOU TREAT A FEMUR FRACTURE IN A 12-YEAR-OLD?

Najeeb Khan, MD
Pradeep Kodali, MD
John F. Sarwark, MD

Children older than 10 years presenting with a femur fracture are generally managed surgically with either internal or external fixation. Acceptable guidelines are more stringent with the older child: up to 10 degrees of varus or valgus, 10 degrees of anterior or posterior angulation, and up to 15 mm of shortening.[1] Rigid intramedullary nailing through the piriformis fossa is not recommended in patients with open proximal femoral physis due to the risk of iatrogenic avascular necrosis of the femoral head, growth disturbance proximally, coxa valga, and thinning of the femoral neck. This risk is diminished once the proximal femoral physis closes.

The indications for external fixation include significant comminution that renders the femur axially unstable, very proximal or distal fractures, subtrochanteric fractures, polytrauma, and significant soft tissue injury such as in open fractures or burns[2] (Figure 22-1). Transverse fracture patterns are poorly suited for external fixation because the small surface area at the fracture site provides less callus and subsequently greater risk of refracture. Pin placement should avoid fracture hematoma, the femoral neck, and the distal femoral physis. Pin track inflammation and superficial infection are common and easily treatable; deep infection is rare. It is important to ensure that the family will be able to perform daily pin-site care with cotton swabs or gauze soaked in equal parts hydrogen peroxide and water.

Flexible or elastic intramedullary fixation using titanium or stainless steel nails is ideal for stable or transverse fracture patterns.[3] Proximal, distal, comminuted, and spiral fractures can also potentially be treated with flexible intramedullary nailing, but may need supplemental spica casting or bracing postoperatively. Flexible intramedullary nailing is

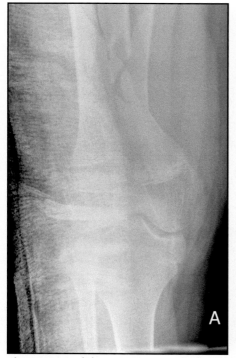
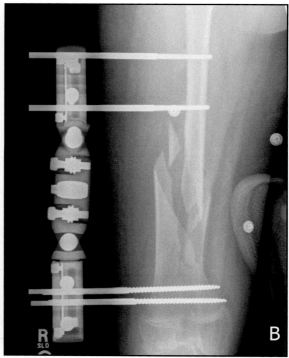

Figure 22-1. (A) Comminuted distal femoral shaft fracture in a 12-year-old not amenable to intramedullar fixation. (B) Two weeks after external fixation. (Case courtesy of Dr. Erik King, Children's Memorial Hospital, Chicago, IL.)

an attractive method because it requires the least amount of management by the patient's family and allows for early rehabilitation (Figure 22-2).

Surgical treatment with flexible intramedullary nails is best done on a fracture table with fluoroscopy. Once traction and fracture reduction is obtained, two C-shaped titanium nails inserted medially and laterally 2.5 cm superior to the physis or one C-shaped and one S-shaped titanium nail both inserted laterally provide three-point fixation within the femur. Preoperative planning should include measuring the narrowest diaphyseal diameter of the femoral canal and then choosing nails that are 40% of the narrowest canal diameter. For example, if the canal diameter is 1 cm, two 4.0-mm nails are used. Each rod should be pre-bent 30 degrees at the fracture site.[4] A drill that is approximately 0.5 mm larger than the nail is used to broach the femoral cortex at an oblique angle that approximates the trajectory of the nail. Once the first nail is just past the fracture site, the second nail can be inserted. Once the nail reaches its final position, it is backed out slightly, cut at the skin, and tapped back in so that only 1 to 1.5 cm lies in the soft tissue.

Postoperative management depends on the fracture pattern. Stable transverse fractures can be placed in a knee immobilizer and made partial weight bearing. A supplemental long leg cast with a derotation bar at the heel should be considered to control rotation in unstable fractures. Generally, transverse fractures can be started on partial weight bearing, whereas oblique or spiral fractures should be nonweight bearing initially.

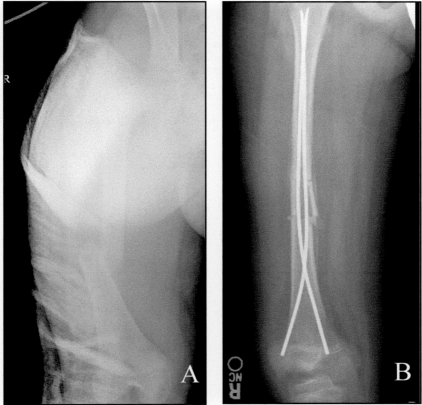

Figure 22-2. (A) Midshaft femur fracture in an 12-year-old in a posterior mold splint. (B) One month after flexible intramedullary nailing. (Case courtesy of Dr. Erik King, Children's Memorial Hospital, Chicago, IL.)

Removal of these flexible nails is surgeon preference. They do not have to be removed, although we generally recommend removal due to concern for future bacterial seeding or hardware problems.

For very distal fractures, flexible nails can be inserted through the greater trochanter. Proximally inserted nails have some disadvantages; later removal can leave a stress riser and there is a possibility of trochanteric apophyseal damage that may lead to coxa valga.

Plate fixation of femoral fractures is rarely used. This method may be considered in cases of concomitant arterial injury requiring vascular repair, very proximal or distal fractures, and in cases of compartment syndrome requiring thigh fasciotomies. Bridge plating, in particular, can be a good option for segmental or comminuted fractures that may also be amenable to external fixation.

Pediatric femoral fractures in this age group generally do well. Flexible intramedullary nailing is an attractive and popular option that allows early rehabilitation and minimal care from the family. The surgeon should consider the risks and benefits of each option as it relates to each patient and his or her family.

References

1. Price CT, Flynn JM. Management of fractures. In: Morrissy RT, Weinstein SL, ed. *Lovell and Winter's Pediatric Orthopaedics.* Philadelphia, PA: Lippincott Williams & Wilkins; 2006.
2. Flynn JM, Schwend RM. Management of pediatric femoral shaft fractures. *J Am Acad Orthop Surg.* 2004; 12:347-359.
3. Anglen JO, Choi L. Treatment options in pediatric femoral shaft fractures. *J Orthop Trauma.* 2005;19(10):724-732.
4. Beaty JH. Operative treatment of femoral shaft fractures in children and adolsecents. *Clin Orthop Relat Res.* 2005;34:114-122.

I Have a 38-Year-Old With a Femoral Shaft Fracture Treated With an Antegrade Nail With No Evidence of Healing 8 Weeks Postop. What Should I Do?

Bradley R. Merk, MD

The treatment of choice for the vast majority of fractures of the femoral diaphysis is reamed intramedullary nailing. The literature is replete with numerous studies reporting union rates in excess of 95% with relatively low complication rates.[1] Uneventful bone healing over the course of 3 to 6 months is the expectation the majority of the time in this clinical scenario. In a minority of patients for a multitude of reasons, however, the normal progression of fracture healing may be altered and result in a delayed union or nonunion. The definition of either is controversial, but I would define a delayed union as a fracture that has failed to heal over the time course anticipated based on the "personality" of the fracture and is at risk for progression to a nonunion or fixation failure in the absence of intervention. I would define a nonunion as a fracture that has failed to fully heal, shows no progression in healing on serial examination, and will not likely heal without additional intervention. Clearly, clinical judgment and experience weigh heavily when making these distinctions and can make formulating a treatment plan difficult.

At 8 weeks after antegrade intramedullary nailing of the femur, solid radiographic union (clear bridging callus on three cortices) is not the rule, but a moderate degree of callus response is expected. In an attempt to formulate a plan in the absence of any significant healing at this point, one must take into consideration a variety of factors to help guide treatment. First, the severity of the bone and soft-tissue injury will have significant impact on the rate of fracture healing. Specifically, one must consider whether the fracture is open or closed, significantly comminuted or simple, and whether or not there are any significant bone defects or actual segmental bone loss present. Second, the condition of the host is also a significant variable. Smokers show slower healing and increased nonunion rates. Patients who are polytraumatized, chronically ill, immunosuppressed, malnourished, and/or noncompliant present therapeutic and healing challenges. Medications such as nonsteroidal anti-inflammatories may also impair healing. In any patient where there is an issue of bone healing, the treating surgeon needs to consider and possibly pursue an infectious workup. Additionally, weight bearing on a nailed diaphyseal fracture of the lower extremity seems to promote healing, and the extent to which this has occurred would influence my expectations with reference to early radiographic healing. Finally, the treating surgeon in the subacute postoperative period must consider technical factors relating to the index procedure. A previous open reduction and the extent to which there may be injury-related or surgery-related periosteal stripping will influence rates of healing. Although less of an issue than in the upper extremity, significant distraction after a statically locked nailing increases the chance of delayed union or nonunion and may prompt consideration of earlier intervention. One should also consider the previously inserted implant. Was there reamed or unreamed insertion? Are the implants of adequate length and diameter to give enough early mechanical stability and withstand the loading that occurs during mobilization in the absence of complete bone healing? Are there adequate interlocking screws present and is there a static or dynamic configuration present? How close is the nail to the knee and how proud is the implant proximally at the insertion point? The answers to these questions will certainly need to be a part of the current and future treatment decisions.

In this patient, I believe that there are five main options to consider for treatment. These include observation, introduction of ultrasound or electric stimulation, dynamization, exchange nailing, or bone grafting. The first option is observation and encouragement of weight bearing. This is a reasonable option if the personality of the injury is such that some impairment of healing was, in fact, expected and the patient is uninfected, able to be mobilized, and pain control is adequate. In addition, the fracture should be well-aligned and stabilized by an appropriately sized nail with adequate interlocking. The patient would need to be clinically and radiographically followed at monthly intervals and if no healing occurred over the next 4 to 8 weeks, I wouldn't hesitate to advocate more aggressive treatment as needed in the near future.

One might consider the addition of noninvasive ultrasound or electric stimulation to the injury in an effort to stimulate healing. These devices are discussed Chapter 47. In general, I would not advocate the introduction of these devices at this time due to a lack of literature support in this clinical scenario.[2] I might consider their use at a later time (4 to 6 months+) in a patient that is a poor surgical candidate and is more clearly headed for or has achieved a nonunion.

Dynamization is a relatively simple procedure to be considered in an effort to stimulate healing. This involves removing interlocking screws from the nail on the opposite side of the isthmus from the fracture to allow axial compression across the fracture site to stimulate healing. Many modern nail designs include a dynamic ovoid hole that allows dynamic compression while maintaining rotational stability. The requirements of this procedure are an axially stable fracture pattern and adequate bone on either end of the nail to avoid significant prominence at the proximal femur or intra-articular protrusion at the knee after screw removal. While appealing as a simple and minimally invasive technique, the support of dynamization in the literature is limited and this is not something that I would routinely recommend at this juncture.[3] The only exception I can envision is if there was a distraction gap of several millimeters at the fracture site after statically locked intramedullary nailing that might compress with dynamization and would not result in unacceptable shortening of the limb or undue rotational destabilization.

Exchange nailing is generally considered a reasonably effective treatment option with high union rates in treating aseptic nonunions of the femur, particularly if the fracture pattern is simple and the comminution is limited.[4] For more complex and comminuted fracture patterns, however, exchange nailing seems to have higher failure rates.[5] In this patient, I would advocate an exchange nailing at this time if the index nail or interlocking screws were of inadequate size to withstand patient mobilization in the absence of healing (Figure 23-1). I would also advocate this treatment in a patient with a relatively straightforward fracture pattern, but with injury or host factors that heavily point towards nonunion risk.

Bone grafting procedures may also be considered in order to stimulate the biology of the impaired healing response in this patient. In this clinical scenario, I would consider an open grafting procedure if there was a reasonably healed and uninfected soft tissue envelope in the presence of an underlying segmental bone defect or significant bone loss following debridement of a severe open fracture. This scenario represents an impending nonunion and should generally be treated aggressively in order to accelerate the patient's healing and return to function.

References

1. Winquist RA, Hansen ST, Clawson DK. Closed intramedullary nailing of femoral fractures: a report of 520 cases. *J Boint Joint Surg Am.* 1984;66:529-539.
2. Busse JW, Bhandari M, Kulkarni AV, Tunks E. The effect of low-pulsed ultrasound therapy on time to fracture healing: a meta-analysis. *CMAJ.* 2002;166:437-441.
3. Wu C. The effect of dynamization on slowing the healing of femur shaft fractures after interlocking nailing. *J Trauma.* 1997;43:263-267.
4. Webb LX, Winquist RA, Hansen ST. Intramedullary nailing and reaming for delayed union or nonunion of the femoral shaft: a report of 105 consecutive cases. *Clin Orthop.* 1986;212:133-141.
5. Weresh MJ, Hakanson R, Stover MD, Sims SH, Kellam JF, Bosse MJ. Failure of exchange reamed intramedullary nails for ununited femoral shaft fractures. *J Orthop Trauma.* 2000;14:335-338.

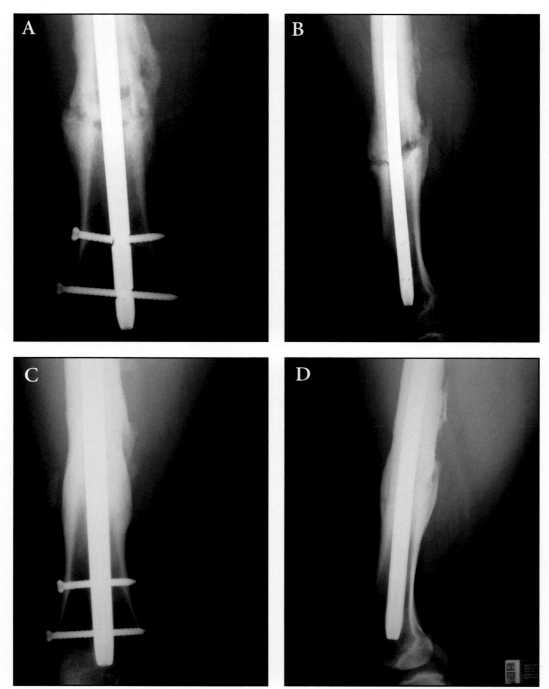

Figure 23-1. A 28-year-old smoker previously treated with an antegrade, reamed, locked intramedullary nail for a closed isolated diaphyseal femur fracture presented with persistent thigh pain during ambulation 6 months after his injury. Preoperative anterior-posterior (AP) (A) and lateral (B) reveal incomplete healing with evidence of interlocking screw fatigue failure. A reamed exchange nailing was performed without formal open bone grafting. The patient was allowed to weight bear as tolerated and his thigh pain abated. Postoperative films at 3 months (C, D) reveal solid radiographic union.

WHAT IS THE BEST TECHNIQUE FOR NAILING A FEMORAL SHAFT FRACTURE IN A 28-YEAR-OLD?

Michael T. Archdeacon, MD, MSE

A femur fracture in a 28-year-old patient will be treated with a statically locked intramedullary (IM) nail. This is the gold standard for treatment of femoral shaft fractures with primary union rates of 96% to 98% and minimal associated complications. In terms of treatment strategy, several issues need to be addressed. First, is this an isolated injury? If so, the patient can be safely managed with IM nailing within 24 hours of presentation. However, if the patient is a victim of multiple injuries (musculoskeletal or otherwise), then the patient may be better served by being moved to a regional trauma center.

Assuming the patient has an isolated injury, the remaining issues revolve around the type of operating room (OR) table required for surgery and the entry portal for intramedullary stabilization. OR table choices include a fracture table to support the limb and provide traction and a flat radiolucent table where manual traction must be applied. Entry portal options include antegrade nailing with a piriformis fossa or trochanteric entry portal, and retrograde IM nailing for some fractures/patients (Figure 24-1).

When considering the type of OR table, one must evaluate the help available. If alone, I would use a fracture table in order to assist with limb manipulation and traction; however, if I have a skilled assistant, a flat-top, radiolucent table requires less set-up time. In either case, care must be taken to avoid rotational malreduction and shortening/lengthening[1]—on the fracture table, lengthening is more likely to occur, while on the radiolucent table, shortening is more likely. It is useful to fluoroscopically measure the nail/femur length on the opposite, noninjured limb prior to initiating the surgery.

In terms of entry portal, antegrade nailing should be considered whenever feasible to avoid violating the knee joint; however, retrograde is perfectly acceptable for many indications. If antegrade is chosen, I would plan a piriformis fossa technique with a percutaneous guide pin or a reverse awl. I prefer the reverse awl because it allows me

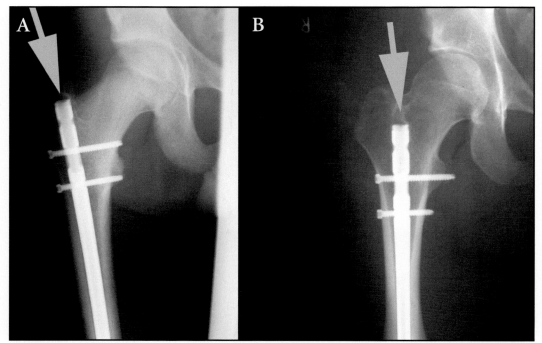

Figure 24-1. Radiographs demonstrating a trochanteric entry portal (A) and a piriformis fossa entry portal (B).

more control for precise placement in the piriformis fossa (Figure 24-2). If the patient is morbidly obese, extremely muscular, or if I have difficulty accessing the piriformis fossa, I would choose the lateral trochanteric entry portal—again, using a percutaneous guide pin or reverse awl.

In terms of benefits and limitations, the piriformis technique is time tested with decades of experience and excellent results. However, the potential of placing the portal anteriorly along the femoral neck is real, and thus the risk of iatrogenic femoral neck fracture must be considered. Additionally, in large muscular patients or obese patients, accessing the piriformis fossa can prove difficult. On the other hand, the trochanteric entry allows for relatively simple access to the femur even in morbidly obese patients. However, the potential for varus malalignment occurs because of the required medial direction of the nail as it enters the canal via the trochanter. This risk can be minimized by rotating the nail so that the anterior bow is directed laterally during nail entry, and then rotating the nail to the appropriate anterior bow as it is passed down the femoral canal. It should be noted that both antegrade techniques will have a detrimental effect on abductor function, and this impairment may persist well after fracture healing.[2]

I use a retrograde technique for patients with morbid obesity and pregnant patients. Additionally, I consider retrograde in the face of concomitant hip or knee trauma, tibial fractures, bilateral femur fractures, and polytraumatized patients. A relative indication for retrograde nailing in my practice is a distal third femoral shaft fracture in which the metaphyseal flair of the distal femur may result in less stability and angular control with an antegrade nail (Figure 24-3).

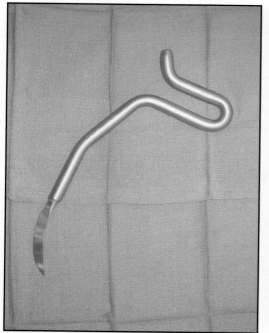

Figure 24-2. Photograph of a reverse awl used to access the proximal femur.

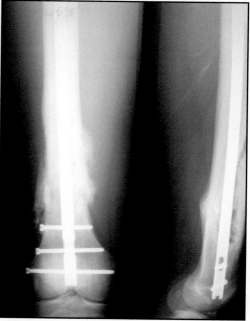

Figure 24-3. Radiograph of a distal third metadiaphyseal femoral shaft fracture treated with a retrograde nail technique.

Once the canal is accessed, closed manipulation of the fracture can usually be accomplished to allow for passage of the guidewire. Care should be taken during reaming to prevent incarceration of the reamer head and excess heat generation. These complications can be prevented by using the reamer at full speed for reaming, advancing down the canal slowly, and increasing the reamer size in half millimeter increments. Of note, the fracture reduction must be maintained during reaming to prevent iatrogenic comminution of the fracture and eccentric reaming that may lead to malreduction. I would advocate a ream-to-fit nailing technique in which the nail placed is one size smaller than reamer size that generated cortical chatter in the isthmus. Ream-to-fit nailing for the retrograde technique yields union rates comparable to antegrade nailing.[3]

Once the nail has been passed across the fracture, the guidewire must be removed, and the reduction should be confirmed both clinically and radiographically. A useful trick for assessing rotational reduction via fluoroscopy involves matching the cortical thickness at the fracture site by gently rotating the distal segment on the nail until the cortical thickness appears equal proximal and distal to the fracture. This technique is obviously limited in the face of extensive comminution. Once acceptable reduction is confirmed, static locking should be performed. I do not recommend locking only proximally or distally (dynamic) because of the potential for loss of reduction with weight bearing. If concerned about axial loading of the fracture, one of the locking screws (proximal or distal) can be placed in a dynamic slot to allow limited axial impaction, but prevent rotational motion. Once locked, the screws should be confirmed within the nail on both AP and lateral fluoroscopy views.

Postoperatively, the patients are allowed immediate weight bearing as tolerated, provided the fracture is within the isthmus region of the femur. Gait training, abductor strengthening, and quadriceps strengthening are initiated on the first day postop and continued as an outpatient for 6 to 12 weeks. I have patients stop formal physical therapy when they no longer exhibit a Trendelenburg gait or Trendelenburg sign and have eliminated their extensor lag. I would anticipate an isolated femur fracture patient to unite the fracture within 10 to 18 weeks postoperatively, but return to manual labor or sports may take 9 to 12 months, depending on the recovery of hip and knee function.

References

1. Wolinsky P, Tejwani N, Richmond JH, Koval KJ, Egol K, Stephen DJG. Controversies in intramedullary nailing of femoral shaft fractures. *J Bone Joint Surg Am.* 2001;83:1404-1415.
2. Archdeacon MT, Ford K, Wyrick J, Paterno M, Hampton S, Ludwig MB, Hewett T. A prospective functional outcome and motion analysis evaluation of the hip abductors after femur fracture and antegrade nailing. *J Orthop Trauma.* 2008;22:3-9.
3. Ostrum RF, Agarwal A, Lakatos R, Poka A. Prospective comparison of retrograde and antegrade femoral intramedullary nailing. *J Orthop Trauma.* 2000;14(7):496-501.

25

I HAVE A TOUGH TIME WITH SUBTROCHANTERIC FRACTURES. ANY TRICKS?

Walter W. Virkus, MD

Subtrochanteric femur fractures are very difficult fractures to treat. There are large muscle forces on the fracture fragments that create significant deformity that is difficult to reduce, and the proximal flare of the femur prevents the nail from "auto-reducing" the fracture. Additionally, the typical abduction deformity of the proximal fragment makes obtaining the proper starting point for an intramedullary nail difficult. Finally, the cortical bone of this region is slower to heal than intertrochantic fractures, leading to late failure in poorly done cases due to the high stresses in this area.

Subtrochanteric fractures result in a fairly typical deformity due to the muscular forces on each fracture fragment. Most significantly, the abductors, iliopsoas, and short external rotators pull the proximal fragment into abduction, flexion, and external rotation, respectively.[1] The adductors and quadriceps lead to shortening. Higher-energy injuries typically have larger fracture displacements and are more difficult to reduce.

Subtrochanteric fractures can be treated by intramedullary nail or open reduction internal fixation (ORIF). Good results are possible with both treatment methods, and there are proponents of each.[2,3] In my opinion, if the fracture can be reduced and the nail starting point is not excessively comminuted, nail fixation is a stronger reconstruction with less operative exposure than ORIF. I reserve ORIF for very short or comminuted proximal fractures.

I prefer to nail subtrochanteric fractures on a fracture table. The reduction is typically much easier if the femur is placed in skeletal traction for the period between injury and surgery. Surgery should be done as soon as the patient is stable, but I try to avoid fixing this fracture in the middle of the night because additional equipment and assistance are often necessary. It is useful to assess the reducibility of the fracture prior to prepping and draping. I set the length and rotation, then manipulate the fracture to be sure I will be able to get it reduced. The tendency to put on more traction is often counterproductive, as it seems to act like a Chinese finger trap and increases the deformity while making it

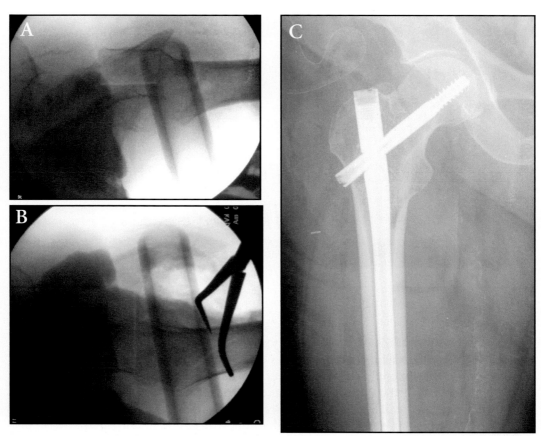

Figure 25-1. Lateral intraoperative fluoroscopic views of a high subtrochanteric fracture after initial traction showing apex anterior angulation (A) and after open clamp application (B). An anatomic reduction was obtained (C).

more difficult to manipulate. Likewise, while it would seem that a crutch under the thigh would help reduce the flexion deformity, it usually simply serves to create a large apex anterior deformity.

It is critical in nailing subtrochanteric fractures that the fracture is held reduced throughout reaming and locking. I get the reduction before doing anything else. I think trying to create the portal in the proximal fragment and manipulate it to pass a guidewire into the distal fragment is a poor approach, as the deformity will recur during reaming. I first use a ball spike pusher through a stab incision in the anterolateral thigh to push the proximal fragment into the proper position. If successful, this is held until the proximal locks are placed. A unicortical half pin can be used in similar fashion. If insufficient assistance is available or this method is not working, I have a very low threshold to open the fracture and place a clamp to hold the reduction. I have not had problems with fracture healing when an open reduction has been done with care. I usually make a 3-inch incision at the fracture site. I make a longitudinal split in the vastus lateralis and push a large pointed clamp against the bone with tines in line with the longitudinal axis. I then rotate the clamp and open it, working one tine around the anterior cortex and one around the posterior cortex. This can almost always be compressed to an adequate or even anatomic reduction (Figure 25-1).

The next critical step in a successful nailing is a proper channel in the proximal fragment. These fractures can be nailed with piriformis or trochanteric starting point nails.[2] The piriformis start can be very difficult due to the abduction of the proximal fragment, particularly in heavy patients. I use a trochanteric entry nail. Although there is a theoretical risk of abductor tendon injury, there have been some as yet unpublished studies that show no significant gait disturbance with trochanteric entry versus piriformis entry nails.

It is critical that a true anterior-posterior (AP) and lateral fluoroscopic view is used when assessing the starting point. This usually means the C-arm must be over-rotated to match the external rotation of the proximal fragment. Likewise, the proper lateral is not with the C-arm parallel to the floor but rotated up slightly. I place the guidewire at the very tip of the trochanteric or just medial. A lateral starting point tends to migrate more lateral with reaming and leads to varus alignment. On the lateral, I assure that the wire is in line with both the femoral shaft and femoral neck so I can place screws into the femoral head if necessary (fracture at or proximal to lesser troch). I then advance the wire so it is in the middle of or slightly lateral in the canal. If the portal is medialized, the proximal femur will end up in varus after the nail is inserted. It is also important that when passing the reamer in and out of the proximal femur, a gentle medial force is applied with the soft-tissue protector to prevent lateral migration of the entry channel. Once the proximal portal is established, reaming is performed while assuring the reduction is maintained. If a trochanteric entry nail is used, the nail should be inserted in 90 degrees of internal rotation so that the anterior bow will curve lateral to avoid impingement of the medial cortex due to the trochanteric entry point. Once the nail is halfway in or so, it is externally rotated to the appropriate position. After the nail is inserted to the correct level, the reduction maneuver/clamp must be maintained until proximal locking is completed.

Although plating seems like an easier way to get these difficult fractures reduced, it is still difficult to manipulate these large fracture segments. When plating subtrochanteric fractures, I prefer to use a proximal femoral locking plate[3] (Figure 25-2). This is easier to place on the proximal segment. The use of the femoral distractor is also very helpful when plating these fractures.

References

1. Russel, TA. Subtrochanteric fractures of the femur. In: Browner B, Jupiter J, Levine A, Trafton P, eds. *Skeletal Trauma*. 3rd ed. Philadelphia, PA: WB Saunders; 2003:1832-1878.
2. Starr AJ, Hay MT, Rienert CM, Borer DS, Christensen KC. Cephalomedullary nails in the treatment of high-energy proximal femur fractures in young patients: a prospective, randomized comparison of trochanteric versus piriformis fossa entry portal. *J Ortho Trauma*. 2006;20(4):240-246.
3. Hasenboehler EA, Agudelo JF, Morgan SJ, Smith WR, Hak DJ, Stahel PF. Treatment of complex proximal femoral fractures with the proximal femoral locking compression plate. *Orthopedics*. 2007;30(8):618-623.

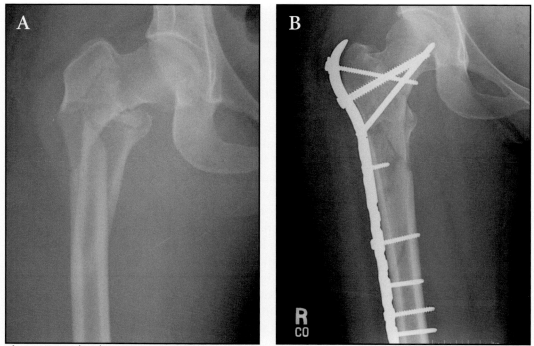

Figure 25-2. (A,B) A comminuted subtrochanteric femur fracture treated with a proximal femur locking plate. The patient's small stature necessitated a slight modification of the standard proximal screw configuration.

WHEN DO YOU USE A SPANNING FIXATOR ACROSS THE KNEE?

Anthony T. Sorkin, MD

The management of complex lower extremity injuries has significantly evolved over the last 10 to 15 years. Rather than forge through lengthy surgical interventions at odd hours in unstable patients, external fixation can provide the surgeon time to adequately assess the injury and allow the patient the opportunity to be appropriately resuscitated. Additionally, it has been shown that immediate open reduction and internal fixation (ORIF) of lower extremity periarticular fractures through compromised soft tissues has higher wound complication rates.[1-3] The theory of damage control orthopedics, therefore, allows for at least partial recovery of the patient's biologic reserve and soft tissues after traumatic injury prior to further reconstructive procedures.[4-6]

There are two categories of patients that, in my opinion, benefit from temporary external stabilization of lower extremity injuries. The first group of patients includes those who are multiply injured or clinically unstable at the time of presentation to the emergency room. I consider any patient diagnosed with a head, chest, or abdominal/pelvic injury with associated long bone or lower extremity injury to be multiply injured and would initiate temporary stabilization. Although this rule cuts a rather wide swath, the only potential harm is overtreatment with a conservative course of action.

The second group of patients that would benefit from temporary external stabilization includes those that are diagnosed with isolated, complex, and unstable extremity injuries with soft-tissue compromise. Frequently, these injuries are associated with shortened, deformed diaphyseal, and periarticular extremity fractures.

Beyond the physiologic benefits discussed above, temporary external fixation for the acute treatment of lower extremity injuries has many additional benefits that are reviewed in Table 26-1. Paramount within that list is the issue of maintaining length to the injured segment, along with obtaining adequate correction of alignment and rotation. Not only does this protect the soft tissues and improve the quality of further radiographic

---

Table 26-1

Benefits of Temporary External Fixation

- Easy to apply
- May be applied rapidly, even with inexperienced staff
- Able to rigidly stabilize multiple, ipsilateral fractures/dislocations during single procedure
- Important in comminuted intra/periarticular injuries to maintain appropriate length
- Significantly improves quality of radiographic evaluation such as CT scan
- Allows easy access to traumatic and surgical wounds
- Minimizes further possible embolic pulmonary insult
- Negligible blood loss
- Patients able to return for definitive fixation when medically/hemodynamically stabilized
- Reduces need for narcotic analgesia
- Improves patient mobility in bed during transfers and with nursing care

---

evaluation, it most importantly and significantly improves the surgeon's ability to obtain an adequate surgical reduction at the time of definitive reconstruction.

The technique used for applying an external fixator across the knee is not complex and can be broken down into two main issues: pin placement and optimizing the stiffness of the fixator for a particular injury. I recommend using non-self-drilling pins with a trocar system to ensure that adequate bicortical purchase has been achieved. There are potential disadvantages related to self-drilling pins such as heat generation and microfracture, but I think that they are much less consequential in the temporary-use setting.

There are specific locations for the pins in both the femur and the tibia. I insert the femoral pins at an angle of about 60 degrees from the horizontal (Figure 26-1). This allows the rectus portion of the quad and the iliotibial band to be spared any further damage. Insertion of the femoral pins at this angle also maximizes the patient's hip flexion and rotation (necessary for comfort while sitting up in bed to eat or log rolled for daily care) even with proximal pins. The tibial pins should be inserted from anterior to posterior just medial to the anterior ridge (Figure 26-2). Because of the triangular shape of the tibia, this orientation will maximize the potential pin/bone interface. The combination of appropriate pin orientations in the femur and tibia is demonstrated in Figure 26-3.

Many of the advantages linked to the use of temporary external fixation are related to obtaining appropriate stiffness in the fixator. Factors that contribute to the need for increasing stiffness include axial instability (severe comminution, segmental injury, unstable dislocation) and the relative distance between the femoral and tibial pins needed to cross the knee. Unfortunately, this is the one aspect of this technique that is easiest to modify and most often overlooked. First, since larger diameter pins lead to increased stiffness, pins of at least 5 mm in diameter should be used in the diaphysis of the femur or tibia. Second, a pin grouping or pin clamp should be used for both the femur and tibia rather than a single pin. This will allow an increase in multiplanar stiffness and the clamps or pin sets can be used as handles to assist in reduction and deformity correction. Next, the pins within the group or clamp should be placed the maximum distance apart. The pin groups or pin clamps should also be placed as close to the zone of injury as pos-

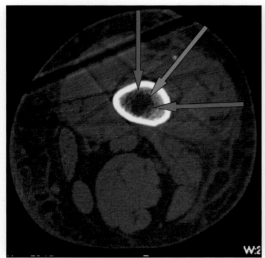

Figure 26-1. Appropriate femoral pin location (green) is anterolateral. Anterior or lateral placement (red) is not preferred.

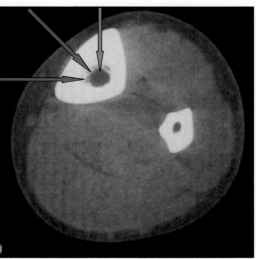

Figure 26-2. Appropriate tibial pin location (green) in anterior. Anteromedial or medial placement (red) is not preferred.

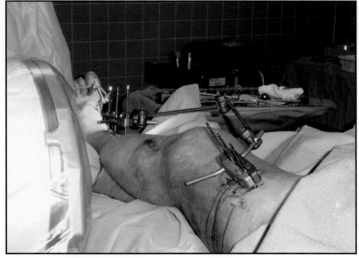

Figure 26-3. Intraoperative photo of appropriate femoral and tibial pin placement.

sible without inserting pins into significantly traumatized tissue. This will minimize the length of the bars crossing the knee and increase stiffness.

External fixation, perhaps more than any other mode of orthopedic intervention, allows for creativity. As a rule, after the initial two bars are applied across the knee, I hold both the femoral and tibial pin clamps and try to deform the injured segment. Any motion that I am able to produce is likely related to the instability of the injury and could further inflame the surrounding soft tissues and be painful for the patient. If I feel that the motion is significant, additional bars or clamps may be applied to increase stiffness and meet the goals of this temporization.

Finally, I recommend extending the frame to the foot in those cases in which the patient is severely compromised (head trauma, ISS >40) or the soft tissue around the

Figure 26-4. Final construct for patient with complex, severely comminuted bicondylar proximal tibia fracture.

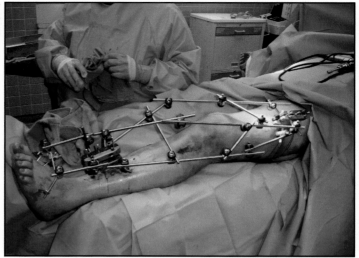

knee is severely threatened (significant fracture blisters, burns, compartment releases). Capturing the foot in the frame early can be the most efficient and safest way to maintain the foot in a neutral position without further potential soft-tissue injury, such as a heel ulcer from an ankle-foot orthosis (AFO). I place two 3-mm pins in the foot, one each in the first and fifth metatarsals. The foot pins are attached to each other with a bar and then combined to the tibial clamp with the ankle held in neutral position. The time for this maneuver is usually less than a minute, but can lead to a big payoff if the patient is otherwise compromised and unable to return for definitive fixation in a timely fashion. Care should be taken in patients at risk for leg compartment syndrome, however, as there is a report that including the foot in the fixator may make diagnosis of compartment syndrome more difficult.

Figure 26-4 demonstrates a temporary external fixator used to initially treat a patient with a comminuted proximal tibia fracture associated with significant ligamentous instability and a second degree popliteal burn.

References

1. Sirkin M, Sanders R, Di Pasquale T, et al. A staged protocol for soft tissue management in the treatment of complex pilon fractures. *J Orthop Trauma.* 1999;13:78-84.
2. Patterson MJ, Cole JD. Two staged delayed open reduction and internal fixation of severe pilon fractures. *J Orthop Trauma.* 1999;13:85-91.
3. Teeny SM, Wiss DA. Open reduction and internal fixation of tibial plafond fractures. Variables contributing to poor results and complications. *Clin Orthop Relat Res.* 1993;(292):108-117.
4. Nowotarski PJ, Turen CH, Brumback RJ, Scarboro JM. Conversion of external fixation to intramedullary nailing for fractures of the shaft of the femur in multiply injured patients. *J Bone Joint Surg Am.* 2000;82:781-788.
5. Scalea TM, Boswell SA, Scott JD, Mitchell KA, Kramer ME, Pollak AN. External fixation as a bridge to intramedullary nailing for patients with multiple injuries and with femur fractures: Damage Control Orthopedics. *J Trauma.* 2000;48:613-623.
6. Pape HC, Giannoudis PV, Krettek C. The timing of fracture treatment in poly-trauma patients: relevance of damage control orthopedic surgery. *Am J Surg.* 2002;183:622-629.

WHAT IS YOUR POSTOPERATIVE MANAGEMENT OF PATELLAR FRACTURES?

Gerald J. Lang, MD

Factors that need to be addressed in the postoperative management of patella fractures include bracing, weight bearing, knee range of motion (ROM), and strengthening of the extensor mechanism.

I generally allow patients with isolated patella fractures to immediately weight bear as tolerated with the aid of crutches or walker. This should be done with the knee in a fully extended position. I also recommend static extension splinting of the knee (with either a knee immobilizer or hinged knee brace that is locked in extension) while weight bearing. Patients can be weaned from crutches as pain allows. In unreliable patients, a cylinder cast (with a pressure relief window over the area of the surgical incision) can be considered. The forces generated across the patellar fracture and repaired retinaculum with contraction of the quadriceps is relatively small when the knee is fully extended. Static extension splinting with weight bearing will minimize the chance of inadvertent knee flexion while the quadriceps is contracting, thus minimizing the risk of fixation failure. This should be continued until the extensor mechanism has healed (generally about 6 to 8 weeks).

My decision making on postoperative ROM varies with the quality of the extensor mechanism repair and the degree of soft-tissue injury about the knee. Fractures with minimal comminution that are stably fixed and have good quality tissues available for retinacular repair are excellent candidates for early ROM (Figure 27-1). Fractures that are marginally stable after repair and have compromised surrounding soft tissue (open fracture wounds or severe soft-tissue swelling) need less aggressive ROM (Figure 27-2). At the completion of the patella fracture and soft-tissue repair, I will assess the competency of the repair. Prior to closure, I will directly inspect the repair by progressively flexing the knee up to 90 degrees. If this is not possible without severely stressing the repair, I consider augmenting the repair by placing a wire or heavy (#5) braided suture looped

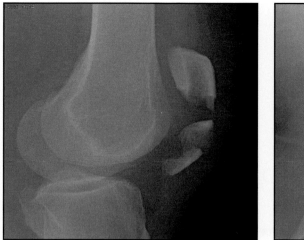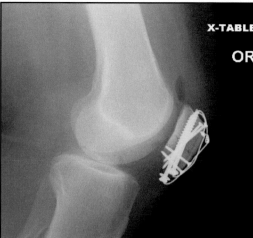

Figure 27-1. Comminuted patella fracture that was repaired in a stable manner and early ROM was instituted.

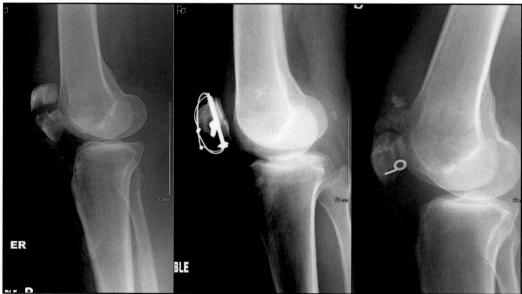

Figure 27-2. Comminuted open patella fracture with severe soft-tissue compromise that delayed attempt at ROM. The perceived quality of the repair was deemed to be marginal. Implant removal and partial patellectomy were required secondary to a delayed infection. These factors contributed to knee flexion of 100 degrees and moderate knee dysfunction.

from the superior pole of the patella to the tibial tubercle, being mindful not to induce an iatrogenic patella baja. This is tensioned to allow 90 degrees of knee flexion.

ROM can commence once postoperative pain is under control and soft-tissue conditions are appropriate. Active, active-assisted, and gravity-assisted flexion can be initiated while sitting on the edge of a table using the uninjured leg to assist in supporting the leg. Heel slides in a supine position can be done as well. Isometric strengthening of the extensor mechanism can commence as soon as comfort allows. With the knee fully extended, the patient can maximally contract the quadriceps muscles and attempt a straight leg raise. Active extension against gravity can also begin in the early postoperative period. As most patella fractures are fixed with some form of tension band construct, some active contraction of the extensor mechanism should generate some compression of the fracture. However, I do not recommend resistive exercises in extension until the extensor mechanism has healed (6 to 12 weeks). Passive ROM to obtain flexion is generally delayed until the fracture and soft-tissue repair are healed. Active and passive ROM are both appropriate to obtain terminal extension. I do not use continuous passive motion (CPM) for postoperative ROM, but this could be employed in certain cases where obtaining a functional ROM may be difficult.

Radiologic evaluation including anterior-posterior (AP) and lateral (and sunrise if possible) views of the knee should be repeated at routine follow-up visits to try to assess whether the fracture is healing (which at times can be difficult) and to make sure that the fixation construct remains competent throughout the rehabilitation process.

The rapidity of return of knee ROM can vary greatly from patient to patient. Fractures that result from high-energy direct trauma to the knee with severe comminution would be expected to regain ROM more slowly. If the patient is not obtaining the desired ROM in a timely manner, there may be contributing factors. If pain is the main problem, the patient may be suffering from an unrecognized complex regional pain syndrome. Occasionally, excessive soft-tissue scarring about the knee can be the main problem. If the patient has not regained a functional amount of flexion (>80 degrees) within 3 months, intervention should be considered. I tend to observe the patient rather than intervene because manipulation of the knee in this scenario would put the patient at risk for rupturing his or her extensor mechanism. I would delay this until the extensor mechanism is fully healed (4 to 6 months). Arthroscopic debridement of the knee could be considered in conjunction with a knee manipulation if intra-articular scarring is considered to be the main cause of stiffness. This puts less stress on the fresh repair. If poor knee flexion is thought to be due to extrinsic scarring of the quadriceps a quadricepsplasty should be considered.

In general, immediate, full weight bearing with the protection of a static extension splint is the mainstay of postoperative patella fracture rehabilitation. Early active and gravity assisted ROM of the knee should be initiated in the early postoperative period if the patellar and extensor mechanism repair and soft-tissue conditions are deemed stable. If these requisites are not present, the ROM will need to be delayed. The degree of pain, stiffness, and overall dysfunction of the limb are often dictated by the severity of injury and the quality of surgical repair. A carefully crafted rehabilitation plan can minimize some of these untoward outcomes.

What Is Your Postoperative Management of Tibial Plateau Fractures ?

George Partal, MD
Marcus F. Sciadini, MD

Our treatment of tibial plateau fractures involves three distinct phases. First, preoperative evaluation involves a complete history and physical exam to identify mechanism of injury, patient comorbidities, and the presence of associated neurovascular injury or compartment syndrome. Radiographic assessment during this phase of treatment routinely includes plain radiographs and computed tomography (CT) scan to accurately define the fracture pattern, degree of intra-articular involvement, and to aid in preoperative planning. The second phase consists of the surgery itself and may include temporizing knee-spanning external fixation in bicondylar fractures or those with excessive soft-tissue swelling and/or fracture blisters. The goals of definitive surgical treatment are to anatomically reduce the articular surface, repair any concomitant meniscal pathology, and provide stable fixation to allow for immediate range of motion (ROM) of the knee. The third phase of treatment is the postoperative therapy and immobilization protocol, which is designed to maximize functional recovery while protecting the soft tissue and internal fixation construct during bony healing. The most common postoperative problems we encounter in treating these injuries are knee stiffness, loss of reduction, flexion contractures, and wound or soft-tissue problems. This postoperative protocol is designed to minimize the occurrence of these problems.

In rare instances, we delay institution of ROM exercises if there are soft-tissue or wound concerns. However, for the vast majority of these fractures, we begin physical therapy for active-assisted and passive ROM immediately postoperatively. Although we think there may be a role for the use of continuous passive motion (CPM) machines in the early postoperative period, we typically avoid their use for a number of reasons. First, we have concerns that the presence of a CPM machine may be seen by nursing staff or physical therapists as obviating the need for formal therapy, which we consider much more beneficial than CPM. Second, ROM readings on the CPM machines tend to overstate the actual motion achieved by the knee due to loose straps and inherent play in the system. Third, CPM machines do not fully extend the knee. We feel that flexion contracture is a frequent complication following tibial plateau surgery and one that is difficult to overcome once it has occurred.

Postoperative immobilization is limited to nighttime use only and for the same reason stated above, we avoid the use of knee immobilizers. These devices tend to allow for mild flexion of the knee, which can lead to flexion contractures. For that reason, we prefer the use of hinged knee braces, locked in full extension, for nighttime use only. Surgical dressings are generally left in place until the initial follow-up visit to minimize exposure of the surgical site to hospital-borne infectious agents. Exceptions include those patients with questionable or at-risk soft tissues whose wounds may be checked at 2 to 3 days postoperatively.

We begin inpatient physical therapy for active-assisted ROM immediately in almost all cases, unless wound issues dictate a short period of soft-tissue rest. Our preferred outpatient physical regimen consists of active-assisted ROM exercises and gentle passive ROM. We find an exercise bike very useful in this early postoperative period. Patients can begin using the bike as soon as comfort allows, long before they resume weight bearing. The seat can be raised to a level that permits the patient to achieve a full revolution and can then be sequentially lowered to increase the knee flexion required. This results in maintaining quadriceps tone and strength as well as some degree of aerobic conditioning until weight bearing can be resumed.

The period of nonweight bearing varies based upon patient factors (age, bone quality, and fracture type), but generally ranges from 6 to 12 weeks.[1,2] We obtain plain radiographs of the knee at the initial follow-up visit (10 to 14 days postoperatively) to assure that there has been no early hardware failure during therapy and usually allow more aggressive passive ROM exercises at this point.

Patients who fail to progress adequately with physical therapy (ie, gaining at least 90 degrees of flexion by 6 weeks), are usually recommended to undergo manipulation under anesthesia.[3] After 8 to 12 weeks, we find that this procedure is much less successful. Those patients that develop significant flexion contractures can achieve satisfactory correction with serial casting if instituted early enough, although a repeat course of therapy to regain flexion is then required.

References

1. Tscherne H, Lobenhoffer P. Tibial plateau fractures. management and expected results. *Clin Orth Relat Res.* 1993;292:87-100.
2. Marsh JL, Smith ST, Do TT. External fixation and limited internal fixation for complex fractures of the tibial plateau. *J Bone Joint Surg Am.* 1995;77:661-673.
3. Weigel D, Marsh J. High-energy fractures of the tibial plateau: knee function after longer follow-up. *J Bone Joint Sturg Am.* 2002;84:1541-1551.

I HAVE A 45-YEAR-OLD FEMALE WITH A BICONDYLAR TIBIAL PLATEAU FRACTURE. WHAT TYPE OF FIXATION SHOULD I USE?

Edward A. Perez, MD

Bicondylar tibial plateau fractures can be of widely varying severity, necessitating a variety of approaches to reduction and fixation. The advent of locked plating has led to a fervor of lateral-based locked fixation in the management of these fractures. Unfortunately, not all fracture patterns lend themselves to a single type of fixation. For all tibial plateau fractures, the basic steps in treatment are:

1. Thorough soft-tissue evaluation and management
2. Anatomic restoration of the articular (joint) surface
3. Stable internal fixation that allows early range of motion

Because many bicondylar tibial plateau fractures are caused by high-energy trauma, injuries to the soft-tissue structures around the knee are frequent. The most important of these are the vascular structures, which should be carefully evaluated before treating the fracture. Any abnormalities in the pulses of the injured extremity should prompt measurement of the ankle-brachial-index (ABI). If the ABI is abnormal (<0.9), immediate vascular surgery consult should be obtained. Compartment syndrome also is common with these fractures, occurring in approximately 20% of high-energy proximal tibial fractures at our institution.

The soft-tissue envelope is often compromised even without vascular injury or compartment syndrome. If the fracture is displaced or length is unstable (shortened), a temporary spanning external fixator is applied. Occasionally, we use a percutaneous screw at this time to reduce the condyles if they remain subluxated even with external fixation. When the soft-tissue envelope permits, open reduction and internal fixation (ORIF) is performed. If the condition of the soft-tissue envelope precludes an open approach, fine-wire external fixation with limited internal fixation at the level of the joint is advisable and has been reported with good results.[1]

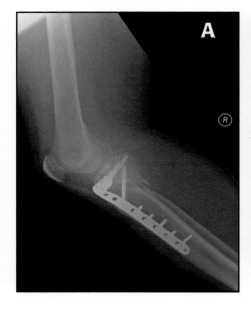

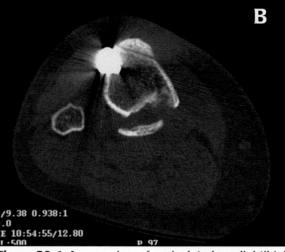

Figure 29-1. A nonunion of an isolated medial tibial plateau fracture treated with a locked lateral plating via a lateral approach without reduction of the medial condyle.

Anatomic restoration of the articular surface with stable internal fixation that allows early functional range of motion is essential to a successful outcome. Critical to the preoperative plan is a computed tomography (CT) scan with the external fixator in place. The CT identifies fracture lines and displacement and helps develop an operative strategy. The choice of approach and implant depends on what needs to be reduced and stabilized. Depressed articular segments must be elevated into an anatomically reduced position before fixation. A "raft" of proximal screws through a plate can be used to support the depressed segment or small-fragment screws can be used when the plate "sits low" on the proximal tibia. As a general rule, a 4.5-mm lateral-based locked plate is the workhorse fixation in this category of injuries. However, lateral-locked plates do not stabilize a displaced medial condyle, and often a medial approach to the proximal tibia is needed to accomplish a medial reduction.

Single versus Dual Incisions and Implants

Historically, bicondylar proximal tibial fractures treated with isolated lateral plating were prone to varus collapse and frequent nonunion (Figure 29-1). However, the soft-tissue complications of single-incision dual plating often were catastrophic. More recently, dual plating through two approaches (anterolateral and posteromedial) has been reported with much lower complication rates,[2] and lateral-based locked plating also has been reported to be successful.[3] The critical question that drives my decision on whether to use a two-incision technique is, "Is the medial condyle reduced?"

There are three general methods for attaining a medial reduction:
1. Nondisplaced medial fracture (no reduction necessary)

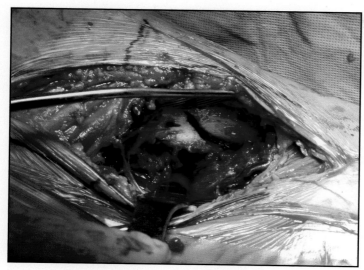

Figure 29-2. A typical appearance of the distal fracture spike (postero-medial tibia) of a medial plateau after a postero-medial approach.

2. Reduced by ligamentotaxis from spanning external fixator or the anterolateral large femoral distractor

3. Direct reduction

If the medial condyle is not displaced or reduces with ligamentotaxis, then the typical fixation I use is a lateral-based locked 4.5-mm plate in conjunction with satisfactory reduction and fixation of the articular surface. In patients with good bone quality, locked screws are not necessary in the diaphysis.

A direct reduction is needed when the medial condyle is displaced and does not reduce through ligamentotaxis. Reducing and securing the medial condyle establishes the appropriate length of the medial side, which makes it simpler to reduce the lateral side to the already stabilized medial column. In essence, a C-type fracture is converted into a B-type fracture (partial articular).

The most frequent position of the distal fracture spike is posteromedial. This finding, in addition to the need to preserve the anteromedial soft-tissue sleeve, makes the posteromedial approach ideal. The interval used is between the pes anserinus tendons anteriorly and the gastrocnemius posteriorly (Figure 29-2). Occasionally, complex fractures require working anterior and posterior to the pes anserinus tendons. This approach allows sufficient access for most medial fractures, while providing a healthy soft-tissue bridge between the two approaches.

The medial fixation does not need to be robust because a lateral plate will be used. For simple fracture patterns, I use a 3.5-mm reconstruction-type plate in buttress mode centered over the apex of the medial fracture line. Occasionally, a small-fragment T-plate is used if more proximal fixation is needed. A medial fracture with a coronal split usually requires reduction with a pointed tenaculum clamp clamp and front-to-back lag screws in addition to a buttress plate. Rarely, two separate plates are necessary on the medial

Figure 29-3. A lateral split fracture with a simple nondisplaced medial fracture stabilized with a lateral locked 4.5-mm plate and lag screw fixation of a nondisplaced coronal split medially.

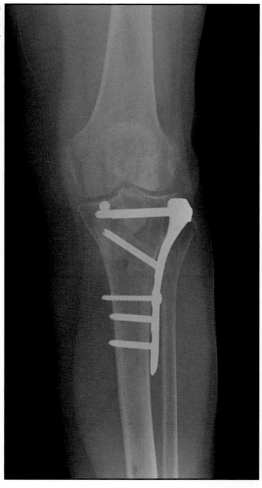

side to achieve the fixation desired. The lateral plate can be 3.5 mm or 4.5 mm, locking or nonlocking, depending on the overall stability needed after reduction.[4]

Frequent Bicondylar Fracture Patterns and Typical Fixation

* Lateral split or split depression with a simple nondisplaced medial fracture (Figure 29-3): lateral locked 4.5-mm plate, with or without 3.5-mm screws to support articular depression.

* Simple articular split with metadiaphyseal comminution (Figure 29-4): lateral locked 4.5-mm plate.

* Lateral split or split depression with a displaced posteromedial fragment (Figure 29-5): medial 3.5-mm reconstruction plate and lateral 3.5-mm periarticular plate

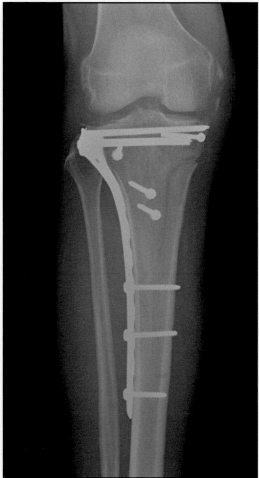

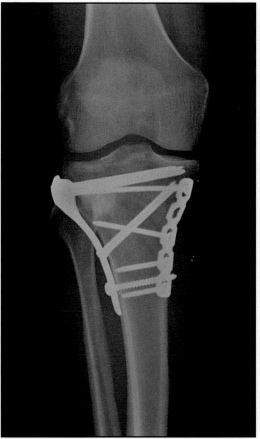

Figure 29-5. A lateral split depression fracture with a displaced posteromedial fragment necessitating a direct medial reduction stabilized with a medial buttress (3.5-mm reconstruction) plate and a lateral periarticular plate.

Figure 29-4. A bicondylar fracture with a simple articular split treated with a locked lateral plate and proximal lag screws for nondisplaced coronal fractures. Additional anterior to posterior lag screws were used to stabilize the tibial tubercle to allow for early range of motion.

✳ Lateral split or split depression with a comminuted medial condyle (Figure 29-6): medial 3.5-mm plate or plates with lag screws and lateral locked 4.5-mm plate

Although the severity of injury to the tibial plateau is strongly associated with the outcome of bicondylar tibial plateau fractures, the treatment goals are the same regardless of the type of injury: appropriate treatment of the soft tissues, restoration of the articular surface, and stable fixation that allows early joint motion. Attaining all three of these objectives provides the best chance for good functional results.

Figure 29-6. Lateral split frcture with a comminuted medial condyle fracture fixed with 2 medial 3.5-mm buttress plates after a direct reduction and lag screw fixation and conjunction with a lateral periarticular plate.

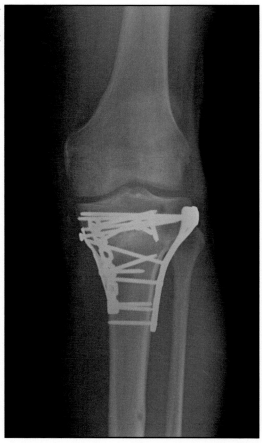

References

1. Rademakers MV, Kerkhoffs GM, Sierevelt IN, Raaymakers EL, Marti RK. Operative treatment of 109 tibial plateau fractures: five- to 27-year follow-up results. *J Orthop Trauma.* 2007;21:5-10.
2. Barei DP, Nork SE, Mills WJ, Coles CP, Henley MB, Benirschke SK. Functional outcomes of severe bicondylar tibial plateau fractures treated with dual incisions and medial and lateral plates. *J Bone Joint Surg Am.* 2006;88:1713-1721.
3. Gosling T, Schandelmaier P, Muller M, Hankemeier S, Wagner M, Krettek C. Single lateral locked screw plating of bicondylar tibial plateau fractures. *Clin Orthop Relat Res.* 2005;439:207-214.
4. Higgins TF, Klatt J, Bachus KN. Biomechanical analysis of bicondylar tibial plateau fixation: how does lateral locking plate fixation compare to dual plate fixation? *J Orthop Trauma.* 2007;21:301-306.

WHAT IS YOUR CRITERIA FOR COMPARTMENT SYNDROME IN THE TIBIA?

James Kapotas, MD

In order to make a diagnosis of compartment syndrome, it is important to incorporate three sources of information: the history, physical exam, and compartment measurements.

Findings in the history that point to concern for a compartment syndrome are a high-energy mechanism of injury such as a pedestrian being stuck by the bumper of a motor vehicle[1]; pain out of proportion to injury; patients who are restless, cannot sleep, or cannot get comfortable due to the pain; or patients whose pain medicine does not relieve the pain. These findings indicate to me that the patient may have a compartment syndrome and further investigation is warranted. If the patient has a head injury, has an altered mental status, or cannot communicate, the only aspect of the history that is usable is the mechanism of injury. By itself, it is not helpful, so you will need to use physical exam and compartment measurement to aid you with your treatment decision.

Physical examination includes sensory, motor, and vascular evaluation, palpation of the compartment, and passive stretching. The first thing I check is the pulse. If the patient has no pulse, it is unlikely that a compartment syndrome caused the loss of the pulse and you will need to rule out a vascular injury in addition to a possible compartment syndrome. I will palpate the tibial compartments and see how tight they are, then check sensation to light touch and see if it is decreased. I check to make sure that the patient can move his or her toes and ankle and if there is pain when moving the toes. I then passively move the toes up and down and see if the patient has pain. If the patient has any abnormal findings on physical exam, I then proceed to compartment measurements.

I use a handheld compartment measuring device. Prior to checking the compartment pressure, it is important to check the patient's blood pressure, know the level of the fracture, and make sure that the leg is not lying directly on the bed, because it can give an artificially elevated pressure in the posterior compartment. I check all four compartments at the level of the fracture, and if needed, do multiple sticks of each compartment. Knowing the pressure at the level of the fracture is important because you can get lower readings further away from the fracture level.[2] If you are concerned about the function of the monitor, you can check the opposite leg for comparison. The criterion for a positive reading is if the compartment pressure is within 30 mm Hg of the diastolic blood pressure.

I divide patients with tibia fractures into four groups:

1. Patients who are alert and oriented, comfortable, and able to sleep. Their neurovascular exam is normal, compartments are swollen but soft, and there is no pain on passive stretch. Clinically, these patients do not have a compartment syndrome and there is no need for compartment measurement. This does not mean that they cannot develop one later—they should be examined within 2 hours to make sure their exam has not changed.

2. Patients who are in extreme pain and cannot get comfortable. Compartments are tight on palpation and they have pain on passive stretch. Clinically, these patients have clear signs of compartment syndrome and need a fasciotomy.

3. Patients are in pain but the pain is controlled very well. Compartments are not tense but they are not soft. They have neurological changes. These are patients in which compartment syndrome is difficult to detect. For these patients, I get a compartment measurement and if it is within 30 mm Hg of the diastolic blood pressure, they will get a fasciotomy. If the measurement is not within 30 mmHg of the diastolic, then I will re-examine the patient in 1 to 2 hours and recheck compartment pressures.

4. Patients who have an altered mental status or are unable to communicate. In this situation, I have a very low threshold to measure the compartment. If the compartments are soft and there are no signs of swelling, then I will not check pressures, but if anything is questionable, I will measure the compartment pressures and proceed with a fasciotomy if the pressure is within 30 mm Hg of the diastolic blood pressure.

It is important to remember that compartment syndrome can evolve and, even though you checked the leg and it did not meet the criteria for a compartment syndrome, it can still develop. It is important that you reexamine patients in 1 to 2 hours, including rechecking pressures if necessary. Continue to check regularly on the patients until they are getting better.

In between checking the patient, it is important to place the tibia level with the heart. Place the patient in a splint and place ice on the extremity; the ice may decrease the swelling and decrease the metabolic demands of the tissue and protect the lower extremity.

References

1. Tornetta P, Templeman D. Compartment syndrome associated with tibial fracture. *J Bone Joint Surg Am.* 1996; 78-A:1438-1444.
2. Heckman MM, Whitesides TE, et al. Compartment pressure in association with closed tibial fractures: the relationship between tissue pressure, compartment and the distance from the site of the fracture. *J Bone Joint Surg Am.* 1994;76-A;1285-11292.

WHAT ARE YOUR TRICKS FOR NAILING PROXIMAL AND DISTAL TIBIAL FRACTURES?

Walter W. Virkus, MD
Ishaq Syed, MD

Proximal and distal third tibia fractures can be challenging. Complications include malalignment, nonunion, and need for revision fixation. Intramedullary nail fixation has become the favored technique for diaphyseal tibia fractures because of superior biomechanics, preservation of extraosseous blood supply, and minimally invasive insertion. Because the metaphyseal flares of the tibia preclude tight endosteal fit of a nail, nail insertion alone does not restore alignment as occurs in the diaphyseal portion of the tibia. There are several "tricks" that allow the surgeon to use a tibial nail in proximal and distal tibia fractures and still achieve stable fixation and acceptable alignment.

Proximal Third Tibia Fractures

Intramedullary nailing of proximal third tibia fractures is associated with coronal (valgus) and sagittal plane (procurvatum) malalignment.[1,2] Factors associated with this malalignment are the patellar tendon extending the proximal fragment and the wide metaphysis of the proximal tibia.[3] To partially compensate for these factors, nailing proximal tibia fractures is usually done through a more lateral starting point. However, this alone is not usually enough to lead to good alignment. A variety of techniques are available but in summary, the fracture must be held in a reduced position during reaming and nail insertion and continue through proximal locking, and the nail must be placed in the proper position.

Figure 31-1. Two-pin fixator used for closed reduction prior to nailing.

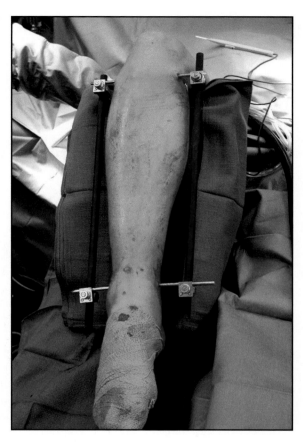

TEMPORARY TWO-PIN EXTERNAL FIXATOR

Temporary two-pin external fixator is our preference for proximal fractures (Figure 31-1). We use 6-mm transfixion pins and place them in the proximal and distal tibia. Proximally, the pin must be kept posterior to the planned path of the nail. Additionally, we use a starting hole in line with the lateral tibial spine, slightly lateral to the standard starting point in proximal fractures. The fixator controls the coronal plane alignment, preventing valgus malalignment, and stabilizes the fracture enough to allow the nailing in hyperflexion. Hyperflexion allows the guidewire to be placed anterior in the proximal fragment, which helps to control procurvatum deformity. If procurvatum persists during nailing, we place a Schanz pin in the proximal segment and use it as a joystick to correct the deformity. The fixator must be left on until the proximal locking screws are placed.

UNICORTICAL PLATE

A unicortical plate can be used as temporary reduction aid and be removed at the end of the procedure at the discretion of the operating surgeon. The plate is typically a 3.5-mm dynamic compression plate placed along the anterior medial cortex to correct both valgus and procurvatum. Unicortical screws should be placed to avoid interference with reamers and the nail.

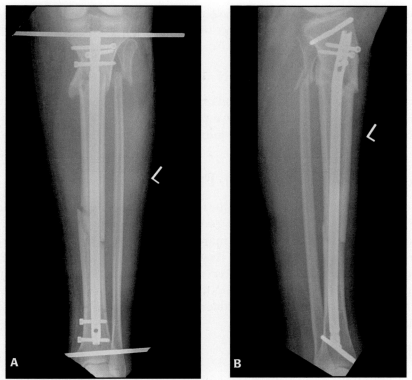

Figure 31-2. Postoperative AP (A) and lateral (B) radiographs demonstrating the use of a two-pin fixator for nailing a segmental fracture.

BLOCKING SCREWS

Blocking screws are placed outside of the desired path of the nail in a strategic fashion to effectively narrow the metaphyseal tibial canal. The screws are placed laterally and/or posteriorly to prevent the standard deformities in proximal fractures. Basically, the screw or screws are placed where you don't want the nail to reside, thus producing better alignment.[2] The locking screws that accompany the nail, or standard 3.5 or 4.5 screws, can be used.

Distal Third Tibia Fractures

Stable distal third diaphyseal fractures can be managed effectively with closed treatment using functional bracing; however, unstable fractures have poor outcome with nonsurgical management and are best treated surgically. The proximity of the fracture to the plafond makes it difficult to achieve stable fixation in the distal fragment, although newer nails with more distal locking holes have extended the ability to nail these fractures. As in the proximal tibia, tight endosteal fit of the nail is not achieved on both sides of the fracture, and as a result the nail alone does not produce acceptable alignment. Both varus and valgus align-ment can be seen.[4] This has led to a resurgence of plating these fractures, particularly with percutaneous methods. The following are techniques for nailing these distal fractures.

PERCUTANEOUS CLAMP FIXATION

Many distal third tibia fractures are spiral or long oblique fractures that can often be reduced with a pointed reduction clamp. We place these clamps under fluoroscopy to minimize soft-tissue disruption. This technique only works with simple, noncomminuted fractures.

TEMPORARY TWO-PIN EXTERNAL FIXATOR

Similar to proximal fractures, this technique is our preference for distal tibia fractures. We place the pins in the same position as in proximal fractures, with the distal pin very distal and anterior in the tibia, as this gives more control over the reduction than placing the distal pin in the calcaneous. While the fixator does an excellent job of maintaining coronal plane alignment, we often have to correct minor translational malalignment by direct pressure using a mallet. It is also important that the reaming wire be perfectly centered in the distal tibia segment. The fixator must be left on until the distal locking screws are placed.

FIBULAR PLATE

Fibular plates are used as a primary reduction aid to help restore length, alignment, and rotation. Studies in a cadaveric model have shown concurrent fibular fracture fixa-tion with intramedullary nailing of the distal tibia fractures reduces angular displace-ment and malunion.

BLOCKING SCREWS

Blocking screws can be useful in preventing malalignment of distal third tibia frac-tures during nailing. The screws can be inserted percutaneously and effectively narrow the width of the metaphyseal medullary canal. Placement is similar to that described for proximal fractures—essentially, screws are placed were you don't want the nail to go, to redirect the nail and facilitate proper alignment.

Conclusion

Surgical fixation of the proximal and distal third tibia fractures can be difficult and requires careful preoperative planning. Many factors are taken into consideration when selecting a type of fixation, including soft-tissue integrity, bone quality, and the frac-ture pattern. Nailing and plating are both reasonable treatment methods in most cases. Regardless of the type of fixation chosen, the goal is stable fixation with proper align-ment.

References

1. Nork SE, Barei DP, Schildhauer TA, Agel J, Holt SK, Schrick JL, Sangeorzan BJ. Intramedullary nailing of proximal quarter tibial fractures. *J Orthop Trauma*. 2006;20(8):523-528.
2. Ricci WM, O'Boyle M, Borrell J, Bellabarba C, Sanders R. Fractures of the proximal third of the tibial shaft treated with intramedullary nails and blocking screws. *J Orthop Trauma*. 2001;15(4):264-267.
3. Buehler KC, Green J, Woll TS, Duwelius PJ. A technique for intramedullary nailing of proximal third tibia fractures. *J Orthop Trauma*. 1997;11(3):218-223.
4. Nork SE, Schwartz AK, Agel J, Holt SK, Schrick JL, Winquist RA. Intramedullary nailing of distal metaphyseal tibial fractures. *J Bone Joint Surg Am*. 2005;87(6):1213-1221.

I HAVE A 38-YEAR-OLD FEMALE WITH A DISTAL TIBIA SPIRAL FRACTURE. SHOULD I TRY TO NAIL THIS OR JUST PLATE IT?

Heather A. Vallier, MD

Spiral distal tibia fractures occur commonly. They are usually an isolated problem, resulting from a low-energy twisting event. Assessment of the fracture and associated soft tissues, in conjunction with discussion of the patient's functional status and expectations, will guide treatment decision making.

Nonoperative management should be considered for minimally displaced fractures or those amenable to closed manipulation and maintenance of alignment with initial casting. Frequently, there is an associated proximal fibula fracture. If the fibula is intact, the likelihood of varus malalignment increases, making closed treatment problematic. The obliquity of the tibia fracture and the degree of adjacent soft-tissue disruption at the time of injury will also influence your ability to maintain a closed reduction. I have a lower threshold for surgical treatment as the obliquity of the fracture increases, because these patterns tend to displace easily, predisposing not only to malunion, but also to irritation of the medial skin at the level of the fracture. Morbid obesity also poses a problem when casting, since it is more difficult to maintain a three-point mold to preserve the reduction.

Angular deformities in the distal third of the tibia cause greater alteration in the ankle joint contact area than more proximal malalignment.[1] One study has shown that tibial malalignment near the ankle produces poor clinical results, with more pain, less motion, and worse degenerative changes over time, compared with more proximal shaft malalignment.[2] These effects were observed with as little as 5 degrees of angular malalignment.

Surgical treatment of displaced distal tibia fractures can improve alignment and provide stability to the bone and the surrounding soft tissues. Stable fixation permits early motion of the adjacent joints and helps to maximize overall function. Treatment options include external fixation, intramedullary nailing, and plating.

Figure 32-1. A plate is inserted through two small wounds, proximal and distal to the fracture, along the subcutaneous border of the tibia. Stab wounds may be placed strategically to introduce reduction clamps or interfragmentary screws.

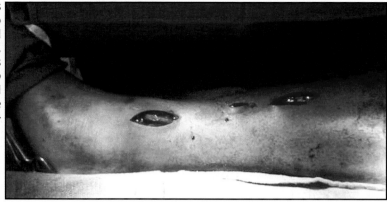

Provisional or definitive external fixation may be warranted for high-energy distal tibia fractures with severe soft-tissue injury; however, external fixation is not warranted for simple low-energy patterns. Compared with other surgical options, it is expensive and poorly tolerated by most patients, with no clear advantage.

Intramedullary nailing has become the standard of care for most displaced tibial shaft fractures. However, proximal and distal shaft fractures can be difficult to control with an intramedullary device, increasing the frequency of malalignment.[3,4] Judicious use of intraoperative reduction aids, such as percutaneous clamps or Schanz screws, will enhance your ability to control these fractures.[5] Recent improvements in nail design with multiplanar distal interlocking options may improve maintenance of fracture alignment after nailing. Studies have indicated that anterior knee pain occurs in up to 57% of patients treated with an intramedullary tibial nail.[6] Meticulous technique, including protection of the patellar tendon, avoidance of the anterior intermeniscal ligament, and placement of an appropriate length nail, may minimize the incidence of knee pain in your patients.

Plate fixation of distal tibia fractures will eliminate the concern of anterior knee pain and decrease the potential for malalignment when compared with nailing. However, plating may devitalize the surrounding soft tissues and bone. Minimally invasive plating techniques reduce surgical trauma and maintain a more biologically favorable environment for fracture healing, reducing risks of infection and nonunion.[7,8] Current literature suggests that plating of distal tibia fractures may be more efficacious in achieving timely fracture union without secondary procedures versus nailing. This may be due to preservation of the medullary blood supply, which is temporarily disrupted with nailing. Underlying patient factors and features of the injury, including fracture comminution, bone loss, and soft-tissue damage also play an important role in fracture healing.

My preference for low-energy spiral fractures of the distal tibia is plate fixation. I frequently insert the plate through small wounds on each end of the fracture, and use the plate to facilitate the reduction (Figures 32-1 through 32-3). Standard large fragment implants work well in this location. One disadvantage is prominence of the plate, which occasionally may result in secondary implant removal.

I reduce and stabilize associated fractures of the medial or posterior malleoli with screws, whether the tibia shaft fracture is treated with a plate or a nail (Figure 32-4). The role of fibula fixation is controversial. I will occasionally stabilize an adjacent fibula

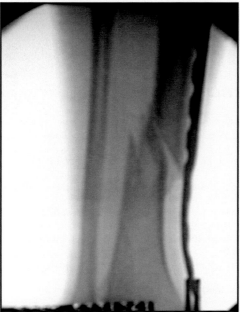

Figure 32-2. Intraoperative anterior-posterior (AP) view demonstrates plate placement along the medial distal tibia.

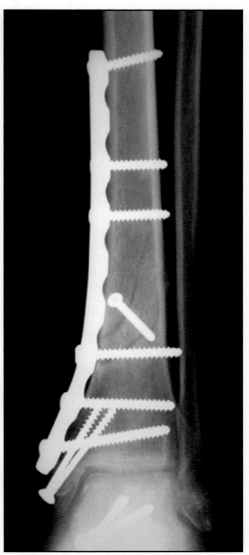

Figure 32-4. Postoperative AP view demonstrating fixation of distal tibia and medial malleolar fractures.

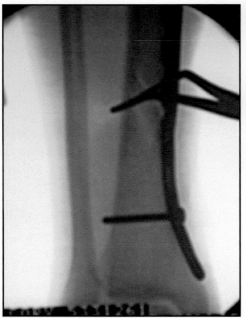

Figure 32-3. Intraoperative AP view demonstrates plate placement along the medial distal tibia (refer to Figure 32-2). The fracture is reduced and clamped, and the plate is secured to the distal segment, facilitating the reduction in antiglide fashion.

fracture. In some cases, the fixation of the fibula will provide lateral stability to the lower leg and facilitate realignment of the tibia. You could also consider fixation for open fibula fractures, or very distal fractures that may adversely affect ankle function.

References

1. van der Schoot DK, Den Outer AJ, Bode PJ, Obermann WR, van Vugt AB. Degenerative changes at the knee and ankle related to malunion of tibial fractures. 15-year follow-up of 88 patients. *J Bone Joint Surg B.* 1996;78:722-725.
2. Puno RM, Vaughan JJ, Stetten ML, Johnson JR. Long-term effects of tibial angular malunion on the knee and ankle joints. *J Orthop Trauma.* 1991;5:247-254.
3. Dogra AS, Ruiz AL, Thompson NS, Nolan PC. Dia-metaphyseal distal tibia fractures-treatment with a shortened intramedullary nail: a review of 15 cases. *Injury.* 2000;31:799-804.
4. Obremskey WT, Medina M. Comparison of intramedullary nailing of distal third tibial shaft fractures: Before and after traumatologists. *Orthopedics.* 2004;27:1180-1184.
5. Nork SE, Schwartz AK, Agel J, Holt SK, Schrick JL, Winquist RA. Intramedullary nailing of distal metaphyseal tibial fractures. *J Bone Joint Surg Am.* 2005;87:1213-1220.
6. Court-Brown CM, Gustilo T, Shaw AD. Knee pain after intramedullary tibial nailing: its incidence, etiology, and outcome. *J Orthop Trauma.* 1997;11:103-105.
7. Oh CW, Kyung HS, Park IH, Kim PT, Ihn JC. Distal tibia metaphyseal fractures treated by percutaneous plate osteosynthesis. *Clin Orthop.* 2003;408:286-291.
8. Redfern DJ, Syed SU, Davies SJ. Fractures of the distal tibia: minimally invasive plate osteosynthesis. *Injury.* 2004;35:615-620.

WHAT IS YOUR
PREOPERATIVE MANAGEMENT OF
A BAD PILON FRACTURE?

Cory Collinge, MD

The goal of surgical treatment for high-energy tibial plafond injuries is to re-establish the articular surface and axial alignment of the distal tibia while allowing for early mobility and predictable healing. Over time, surgeons have realized that they must account for the significant soft-tissue damage commonly associated with this type of injury. Without thoughtful consideration of the soft tissues, disastrous soft-tissue complications may occur in half or more of high-energy tibial plafond fractures treated with open reduction and internal fixation (ORIF). The anatomy of the leg is particularly susceptible to soft-tissue complications because the distal tibia and fibula are contained within a relatively delicate soft-tissue envelope and are supplied by a limited vascular network compared to other parts of the extremities.

A thorough and meticulous examination is important in the evaluation of patients with these high-energy fractures. All associated injuries must be identified and formulated into the treatment plan; 5% to 10% of plafond fractures are bilateral, 30% have ipsilateral lower extremity injuries, and 15% have injuries to the spine, pelvis, or upper extremities. Approximately 20% to 40% of plafond fractures are open, reflecting the severity of the injury and the necessity for aggressive soft-tissue management. Open fractures must be treated with immediate administration of appropriate antibiotics, a moistened saline dressing, and splinting. Urgent and thorough surgical debridement is standard, and I usually combine this with fracture stabilization using external fixation (Figures 33-1 and 33-2). In selected cases, fixation of the articular injury may be best performed at this setting, as articular exposure may be optimal (Figure 33-3). Certainly, the surgeon must be comfortable that the fracture site is "clean" to proceed in this manner, but later reconstruction may be made more simple and perhaps less invasive.

Teeny and Wiss[1] and McFerran et al[2] both showed that early ORIF of high-energy plafond fractures can have both poor early results and disastrous eventual outcomes, with

Figure 33-1. Injury radiographs of 43-C3 fracture demonstrating deformity including significant shortening and malalignment.

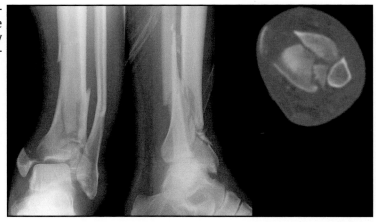

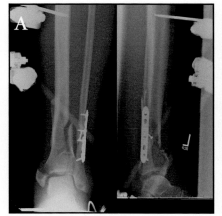
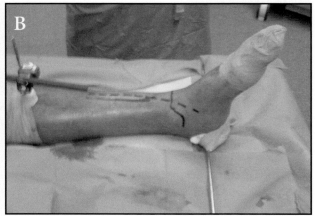

Figure 33-2. (A) After stabilization with fibular plating and external fixator, alignment is much improved and the joint is decompressed. No further harm will likely occur and soft tissues may recover with time and elevation. (B) Return to surgery for reconstruction occurs when the soft tissues are quiescent.

major complication rates of 40% to 50%. These poor results with early open treatment appear primarily related to the disruption of the soft-tissue envelope, not the fixation of the bony fracture itself.

The complexity of these injuries considered, the past decade has witnessed the development and widespread acceptance of treatments that emphasize soft-tissue damage control, including temporizing external fixation and staged reconstruction. Sirkin et al[3] and Patterson and Cole[4] similarly reported a staged protocol for management of high-energy injuries with early stabilization of the fibula fracture and temporary spanning external fixation of the tibia across the ankle joint (see Figures 33-2 and 33-3). Formal open reconstruction of the tibial plafond with open plating was performed when soft tissues normalized (mean 13 and 24 days, respectively). Using this approach, Sirkin et al[3] found only 3 deep infections in 56 cases (6%) and Patterson and Cole[4] found none in 22 cases. No other major complications were seen. Generally, most experts agree that swelling and edema should be controlled before surgery is undertaken in order to minimize the risk of soft-tissue complications. Marked swelling, the presence of fracture blisters, or other skin

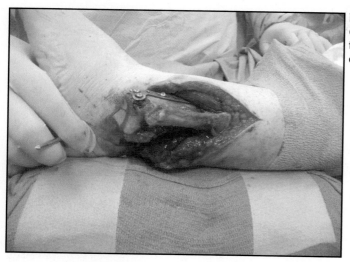

Figure 33-3. In some extreme cases, articular reconstruction of the plafond can be performed early through the open wounds.

changes should delay surgery until the soft tissues have had time to recover. If this is the case, the fracture is probably best treated in a staged fashion with early external fixation and delayed reconstruction.

If the staged protocol is to be used, consider whether the fibula can be anatomically reduced and fixed. If the surgeon is not certain that he or she can make the fibula "perfect," then the fibula should not be addressed initially. The external fixator can be applied, adequate gross reduction of the talus beneath the tibia obtained with traction, and the fibula left for the definitive surgery. If the fibula is to be addressed, moving the skin incision posterior by 1 to 1.5 cm may help avoid some soft-tissue problems and allow more options for approaches at the time of final reconstruction.

I use a simple external fixation construct linking the tibial diaphysis (proximal to area of proposed plate placement) to the calcaneus for the temporary fixator. The patient is discharged with instructions for elevation and restricted daily activities while awaiting soft-tissue improvement. The patient should return at regular intervals between 5 days and 2 to 3 weeks after injury to schedule and undergo definitive tibial internal fixation. The return of skin wrinkles, blister epithelialization, and improvement in ecchymosis are several parameters to observe when staging the open procedure. In most cases, the external fixation is removed after internal stabilization, but pins can be incorporated into the preparation and drape and used intraoperatively with a femoral distractor (or ex fix) for obtaining reduction and provisional stabilization of the articular surface.

Preoperative planning for definitive plafond treatment can often minimize delays during the surgery and allows the surgeon to make errors "on paper" instead of in the operating room. A good preoperative plan can help with choosing the optimal surgical approach (including patient positioning), preferred reduction methods, implant selection and placement, bone graft needs, and other treatment needs. Part of the preoperative plan for these injuries is quality radiographs of the ankle and a computed tomography (CT) scan.

In summary, high-energy tibial plafond fractures are complex injuries that have a high potential for complications if not managed thoughtfully. As many of these complications are somewhat preventable, tibial plafond fractures present the orthopedic surgeon with a real opportunity to influence a patient's ultimate outcome. While we cannot alter the severity of a particular injury, appropriate surgical timing and soft-tissue handling, along with exact articular reduction and stable fixation to allow for early motion, offer the best chance of obtaining good results with few complications for patients with these fractures.

References

1. Teeny SM, Wiss DA. Open reduction and internal fixation of tibial plafond fractures. Variables contributing to poor results and complications. *Clin Orthop.* 1993;292:108-117.
2. McFerran MA, Smith SW, Boulas HG, et al. Complications encountered in the treatment of pilon fractures. *J Orthop Trauma.* 1992;6:195-200.
3. Sirkin M. Sanders R, DiPasquale T, et al. A staged protocol for soft tissue management on the treatment of complex pilon fractures. *J Orthop Trauma.* 1999;13:78-84.
4. Patterson MJ, Cole JD. Two-staged delayed open reduction and internal fixation of severe pilon fractures. *J Orthop Trauma.* 1999;13:85-91.

HOW DO YOU DECIDE WHICH SURGICAL APPROACH TO USE FOR PILON FRACTURES?

Jeffrey M. Smith, MD
Anthony G. Sanzone, MD

In order to achieve a successful outcome in treating pilon fractures, proper decision making regarding timing of surgery, approach, and implant selection are all critical. It is well-documented that the proper handling of the soft tissues around the ankle joint is paramount.[1] Upon initial evaluation of most pilon fractures (except perhaps those with minimal displacement or an extremely low-energy mechanism), we apply a spanning external fixator in an urgent fashion. Various constructs for the fixator can be performed. Specifically, two anteromedial Schantz pins are placed in the tibia and one in the calcaneus. It is reasonable to place a supplemental pin in the first metatarsal base or to use the talus instead of the calcaneus, but this is not our preference. Regardless of the construct used, it is critical that the pins are well outside the field where one will make the appropriate incision during the next stage.

Stabilizing the fibula can then be considered. If fibular stabilization is to be performed, it should be done within the first 24 hours or there will be significant difficulty closing the incision. In addition, fibular stabilization should only be attempted when the treating surgeon is confident that the appropriate alignment of the fibula (proper length and rotation) can be successfully restored. If the fibula is too comminuted, fracture reduction and alignment are frequently suboptimal, which will interfere with anatomic reduction of the tibial pilon. In addition, we use a posterolateral approach to the fibula to allow an appropriate skin bridge for the second-stage procedure or leave the fibula unfixed to avoid problems with the above issues and maintain the option of a second-stage anterolateral or direct lateral approach.

Although it is favorable to anatomically reduce and internally stabilize these fractures, there are several host factors that lead us to consider spanning external fixation (potentially with a hybrid construct) with or without limited internal fixation. These include

Figure 34-1. Anterior approach to tibial pilon demonstrated with additional markings for the anterolateral and anteromedial approaches. Classically, the tibialis anterior is retracted medially for the anterior approach, but it would be retracted laterally for an anteromedial approach.

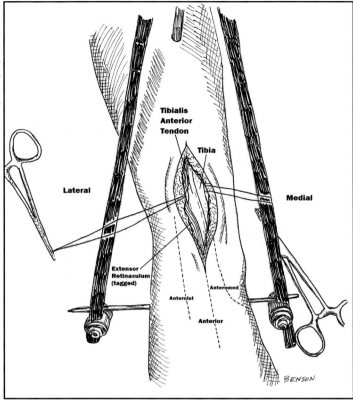

smoking, diabetes, chronic steroid use, patient age, severe osteoporosis, and rheumatoid arthritis. In patients with these or multiple comorbidities, we even consider nonoperative treatment.

Timing of the second stage of the procedure is dictated by the integrity of the soft tissues. We prefer to drain and apply Silvadene cream (Aventis Pharmaceuticals Inc, Paris, France) to fracture blisters and initiate routine fixator pin care. Once fracture blisters have re-epithealized, swelling has subsided, and skin wrinkling is apparent (usually 7 to 21 days), definitive stabilization may be performed. After first stage treatment, radiographs and computed tomography (CT) scanning are essential for definitive stage preoperative planning and will dictate our approach. Numerous anatomic implants specifically designed for the tibial plafond are now available and should be exploited.

The standard approaches to the tibial pilon include anterior, anterolateral, direct lateral, posterolateral, direct medial, anteromedial, and posteromedial.[2] The primary determinant for choosing a surgical approach is access to obtain the reduction of the major articular fragments, while the secondary factor is the placement of hardware that will best support and maintain the reduction. Usually, the direction of greatest displacement (shortening) and angulation will guide the surgeon, such that anterolateral or anterior impaction (apex posterior angulation) is best approached from either anterior (Figure 34-1) or anterolateral (Figure 34-2), and posterior shortening (apex anterior angulation) is best approached posterolateral or posteromedial. Varus angulation can be addressed through any of the medial approaches, but it is more likely to have symptomatic hardware if placed medi-

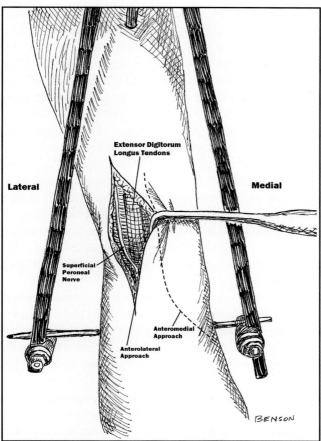

Figure 34-2. Anterolateral approach to tibial pilon. The superficial peroneal nerve should be identified and protected throughout the reconstruction. The extensor digitorum longus and peroneus tertius are retracted medially to expose the distal tibia.

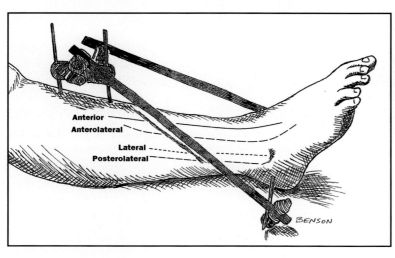

Figure 34-3. Lateral view of the ankle demonstrating the various skin incisions for the tibial pilon. The anterolateral, direct lateral, and posterolateral also allow access to the fibula for reconstruction.

ally. The anterolateral and posterolateral approaches (Figure 34-3) allow additional access to the fibula through the same incision. The anteromedial approach allows access to the anterior pilon and the medial malleolus fragment through the same incision, but it is more prone to wound healing complications with exposed bone or hardware.

Direct visualization of the articular surface can be enhanced by using the fixator as a distractor or by removing the external fixator, placing a Schantz pin in the talus, and placing the femoral distactor on both a remaining tibial pin and the talar pin. The primary goal of surgery is anatomic articular reduction,[3] and we usually prefer to reconstruct the pilon from a posterolateral to anteromedial manner. Articular reconstruction is initially held with multiple k-wires placed in strategic locations, thereby not interfering with definitive stabilization nor stretching skin edges. Cancelleous allograft chips or various bone substitutes are commercially available to provide structural support in areas of bone defects and potentially encourage osteoconduction. Combined approaches are occasionally needed to achieve anatomic reduction and adequate rigid stabilization. We try to maintain a skin bridge of at least 5 cm, while coordinating access to the major articular fragments for reduction and fixation, such as anterolateral with posteromedial, direct medial with direct lateral, anteromedial, and posterolateral. Protection of skin edges is maximized by avoiding excessive undermining and traction to skin edges, and we select implants that minimize hardware prominence. When feasible, percutaneous plating techniques help limit skin incision damage. Wounds are closed under minimal tension over a small hemovac drain using a Donati type stitch.

Open fractures also pose a significant challenge. In addition to the aforementioned principles and emergent debridement and irrigation, consideration for immediate open reduction and internal fixation (ORIF) can be made with subsequent soft-tissue coverage contingent on the size and contamination of the wound. Osteochondral fragments without soft-tissue attachment need to be thoroughly debrided, retained, and at least provisionally stabilized. Plastic surgery consultation is initiated early to determine a strategy for soft-tissue coverage, be it skin grafting, local flap, or free flap coverage. While we prefer primary wound closure or early flap coverage, wound VAC application can be used as a temporizing method for wound closure. Liberal use of antibiotics is suggested in these potentially limb-threatening injuries.

References

1. Whittle P, Wood GW II. Fractures of lower extremity. In: Canale T, ed. *Campbell's Operative Orthopaedics.* 10th ed. St. Louis, MO: Mosby; 2003:2741-2750.
2. Masquelet AC, McCullough CJ, Tubiana R, Fyfe IS, Klenerman L, Letournel E, eds. *An Atlas of Surgical Exposures of the Lower Extremity.* London: Taylor and Francis; 1993:214-239.
3. Stephen DGJ. Fractures of the distal tibial metaphysis involving the ankle joint: the pilon fracture. In: Schatzker J, Tile M, eds. *Rationale of Operative Fracture Care.* 3rd ed. Berlin: Springer; 2005:523-550.

DO YOU TAKE OUT SYNDESMOTIC SCREWS IN ADULT PATIENTS?

Joseph D. DiCicco, DO
Micah C. Hobbs, DO
Matthew W. Heckler, DO

Ankle fractures are one of the most common injuries treated by orthopedic surgeons. Managing associated injuries to the distal tibiofibular syndesmosis is often difficult. The evaluation of syndesmotic injuries can be a challenge, and considerable controversy exists regarding the optimal method of fixation, including screw size, number of cortices required for screw purchase, the role of bioabsorbable implants, weight bearing status postoperatively, and the need for and timing of syndesmotic screw removal. Despite this controversy, timely identification and stable internal fixation are necessary for proper management of syndesmotic injuries.

The tibiofibular syndesmosis is composed of the anterior tibiofibular, posterior tibiofibular, transverse tibiofibular, and interosseous ligaments. The posterior tibiofibular ligament is the primary restraint to posterolateral displacement of the fibula.[1] A variety of clinical and radiographic signs can confirm the presence of syndesmotic disruption. Clinical signs of injury include pain associated with compression of the distal tibia and fibula, pain with external rotation of the ankle, and tenderness to palpation localizing over the syndesmosis. Patients with proximal fibula pain should have appropriate radiographs taken to rule out Maisonneuve fracture.

Fibula fracture associated with medial joint space widening indicates an unstable ankle and should raise suspicion for disruption of the tibiofibular syndesmosis.[2] Standard static radiographic views indicate syndesmotic disruption by measuring greater than 5 mm of clear space between the tibial incisura and medial border of the distal fibula. As external rotation forces are the primary mechanism of injury to these ligaments, syndesmotic disruption is typically seen with Weber C and pronation-external rotation type patterns. However, disruption is also commonly seen in supination-external rotation injury patterns because the level of fibula fracture cannot accurately predict syndesmotic integrity.[2,3] In fact, dynamic instability of the syndesmosis can occur without associated fracture in patients with a "high ankle sprain." Stress radiographs can be taken with an external rotation force applied to the ankle. An increased clear space or the presence of medial joint space widening secondary to lateral talar shift and external rotation of the fibula indicates syndesmotic disruption.

Intraoperative assessment can be made by applying a direct lateral pulling stress to the distal fibula (Figures 35-1A and 35-1B). Syndesmotic instability is indicated by greater than 1 cm of tibiofibular separation or by widening of the medial clear space.[2] However, posterior displacement of the fibula with external rotation of the ankle has been shown to be a more reliable indicator of syndesmotic injury.[1] Overall clinical impression, based on a combination of the subjective and objective signs described above, is the best indicator to predict syndesmotic ligament disruption.

Anatomic reduction of the fibula within the tibial incisura is our goal (Figures 35-1C and 35-1D) Use of percutaneous reduction clamps without direct visualization of the syndesmosis is often used, but may lead to a nonanatomic reduction. Open reduction allows direct visualization and accurate restoration of preinjury anatomy. The position of the foot during syndesmotic stabilization has not shown to affect postoperative range of motion (ROM).[4]

Stable fixation can be accomplished with a variety of implants. While comparative studies have not demonstrated a superior technique, screw fixation of three or four cortices with 3.5-mm or 4.5-mm cortical screws has proven to be effective. We prefer using a 3.5-mm cortical screw engaging three cortices. Engaging the lateral tibial cortex only allows physiologic motion to occur between the distal tibia and fibula once weight bearing is allowed. Advancing the syndesmotic screw to engage the medial tibial cortex may decrease the risk of late tibiofibular diastasis, but is associated with the increased risk of hardware failure when weight bearing resumes.[2] Bioabsorbable screws have been used to stabilize the syndesmosis and early results show it is a dependable treatment alternative.

Postoperative management of the syndesmosis remains controversial. Classically, patients are nonweight bearing for 8 to 12 weeks, depending on surgeon satisfaction with fixation. We begin guided physical therapy immediately after stabilization of the syndesmosis to restore ankle ROM. We typically perform screw removal in the operating room at 8 weeks and progress weight bearing at that time. All patients are stressed under fluoroscopy in the operating room to determine syndesmotic stability at the time of screw removal. We agree that screw removal may reduce syndesmosis stiffness and eliminates the risk of intramedullary screw breakage.[2] While late diastasis after screw removal has been documented, we have not found this to be an issue using our protocol.[3] Screw removal may be performed in the office for select patients. Limited hardware removal in the office prevents subjecting your patient to multiple episodes of general anesthesia, is more cost-effective than returning to the operating room, and has shown to be well-tolerated in a similar case series.[5] Ultimately, successful management of the distal tibiofibular syndesmosis requires an accurate diagnosis, anatomic reduction, stable fixation, and a postoperative protocol that avoids complication.

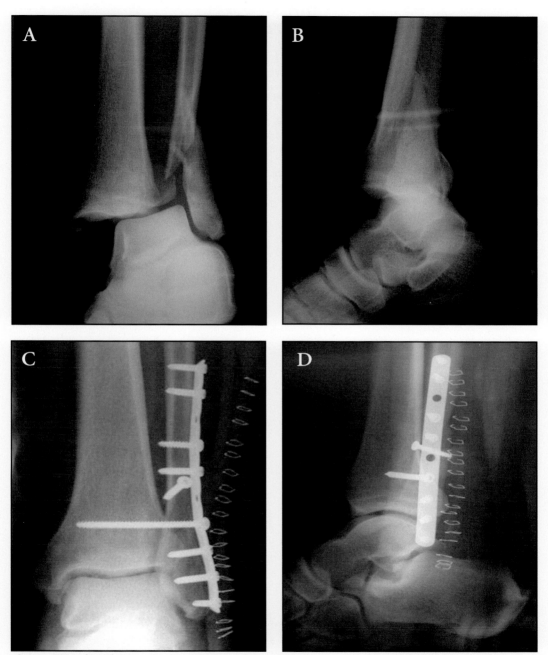

Figure 35-1. (A, B) Trimalleolar fracture-dislocation of tibiotalar joint. Syndesmotic disruption confirmed intraoperatively. (C, D) Postoperative films demonstrate stabilization using 3.5-mm cortical screw through a one-third tubular locking plate with tricortical purchase.

References

1. Xenos JS, Hopkinson WJ, Mulligan ME, Olson EJ, Popovic NA. The tibiofibular syndesmosis. Evaluation of the ligamentous structures, methods of fixation, and radiographic assessment. *J Bone Joint Surg Am.* 1995;77(6):847-856.
2. Vander Griend R, Michelson JD, Bone LB. Fractures of the ankle and the distal part of the tibia. *Instr Course Lect.* 1997;46:311-321.
3. Nielson JH, Sallis JG, Potter HG, Helfet DL, Lorich DG. Correlation of interosseous membrane tears to the level of the fibular fracture. *J Orthop Trauma.* 2004;18(2):68-74.
4. Tornetta P 3rd, Spoo JE, Reynolds FA, Lee C. Overtightening of the ankle syndesmosis: is it really possible? *J Bone Joint Surg Am.* 2001;83(4):489-492.
5. DiCicco JD, Ostrum RF, Martin B. Office removal of tibial external fixators: an evaluation of cost savings and patient satisfaction. *J Orthop Trauma.* 1998;12(8):569-571.

I Have a Male Patient With a Trimalleolar Fracture, But the Posterior Malleolus Is Minimally Displaced. Do I Need to Fix It?

Rajeev Garapati, MD

Posterior malleolar fractures occur in approximately 7% of ankle fractures.[1] They are usually caused by tensile forces applied through the posterior inferior tibial fibular ligament (PITFL), but can also be caused by compressive forces applied through the talar dome. The fragment is usually posterolateral, but axial loading or supination-adduction ankle fractures can cause a more medial portion of the posterior lip to fracture.[2]

It is important to recognize that there is a posterior malleolar fracture fragment and to accurately characterize its size, shape, and location. This can be very difficult to do on initial x-rays where the ankle is subluxated or dislocated. Getting a provisional reduction and appropriate postreduction x-rays can help facilitate the evaluation. The posterior malleolar fragment often is seen as a "double density" on the anterior-posterior (AP) or mortise x-ray. An external rotation lateral view, performed by placing the x-ray beam parallel to the fracture line, can better delineate the posterior malleolus and can be very useful in the evaluation of this difficult-to-visualize piece.[3] If there is any uncertainty regarding the posterior malleolus, a preoperative computed tomography (CT) scan is warranted. Transverse (axial) CT scan images provide information regarding the size, location, comminution, and displacement of the posterior lip.

The major effects of a posterior malleolus fracture are increased rotational instability and posterior subluxation of the talus in the mortise.[4] Occasionally, with large posterior malleolar fractures in conjunction with fibula fractures, there is such instability that the talus cannot be held reduced in the mortise. Dorsiflexion tends to make the situation worse by tightening the posterior myotendinous units. The amount of instability in posterior malleolus fractures depends on whether the lateral structures are intact. With intact lateral structures, posterior stability is maintained even with a 50% defect in the posterior malleolus.[4]

Indications for fixing a posterior malleolus fracture are often unclear and ambiguous. Commonly cited indications are for fractures that involve >25% to 35% of the distal tibial articular surface or for fractures that have >2 mm to 3 mm of displacement after fixation of the medial and lateral malleolus. Other indications include fractures with posterior subluxation of the talus or to help stabilize the syndesmosis by restoring the integrity of the PITFL.[1] In any regard, the indication to fix a posterior malleolus is up to the judgment of the surgeon.

The technique for reduction and fixation depends on the size and location of the fragment and the incisions required for the associated components of the fracture. A direct approach can be done when there is a large posterior malleolar fragment (>30% to 40% of the articular surface) or one in which there is some posterior malleolar comminution. This can be done with the patient prone or with a large bump under the hip to place the patient in a semi-lateral position. For posterolateral fragments, the approach is between the Achilles and peroneal tendons. The incision is posterolateral, which allows for access to both the posterior malleolus and the fibula. You must watch for and protect the sural and superficial peroneal nerve during the approach. For posteromedial fractures, the approach is from the medial side with retraction of the flexor tendons and neurovascular bundle. The joint cannot be visualized through either posterior approach and thus, the reduction is assessed by extra-articular fracture lines, usually the proximal spike. Fixation options include lag screws, usually 3.5-mm cortical or 4.0-mm cancellous, or a buttress (antiglide) plate in addition to lag screws, depending on the exposure and size of the fragment.

More commonly, indirect reduction and fixation is performed. Reduction of the medial and lateral malleolus is done with standard techniques and then the posterior malleolus is evaluated. Anatomic reduction of the fibula will lead to an indirect reduction of the posterior malleolus through the intact posterior tibial fibular ligaments. If there is any indecision regarding the need to fix the posterior malleolus, now is the time to decide. If there is any posterior subluxation, if the piece is larger than 30% of the articular surface, or if there is significant (>2 mm) displacement, then it should be fixed. One should also do a posterior drawer test and if the talus subluxates posteriorly, then the posterior malleolus should be fixed. If none of the above exist, one can proceed with nonoperative treatment.

If the decision has been made to proceed with fixation, the reduction must first be checked fluoroscopically. It can be adjusted with a percutaneous tenaculum clamp if needed. Fixation is then performed from anterior to posterior. This is usually done with two 4.0-mm partially threaded cancellous screws. You must be sure, however, that the posterior malleolus fragment is large enough so that all the threads cross the fracture site, otherwise you will not achieve interfragmentary compression. If the posterior malleolus fragment is small, then it is better to use standard lag technique with 3.5-mm cortical screws. It is ideal to put the screws close to the joint because the posterior malleolus is larger at that level. You also want to be perpendicular to the fracture line; thus, the screws are usually angled slightly anteromedial to posterolateral. The reduction and fixation is confirmed fluoroscopically.

In summary, there is still much controversy regarding the ideal treatment of trimalleolar fractures. Each patient and case must be evaluated individually. A thorough understanding of the mechanism of injury and the role of the posterior malleolus is necessary

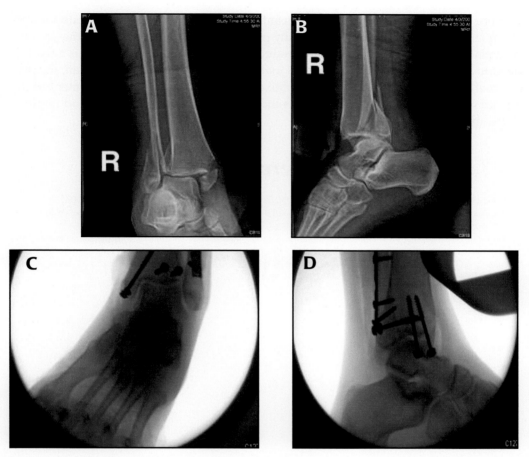

Figure 36-1. Mortise (A) and lateral (B) radiographs of a trimalleolar ankle fracture with a significant posterrior malleolus fracture. Posteroperative mortise (C) and lateral (D) fluoroscopic views demonstrating fixation including posterior to anterior screws stabilizing the posterior malleolus.

to achieve an optimal outcome. For significantly displaced or comminuted posterior malleolar fractures, the best approach is usually posterior. For smaller fractures, the decision can be made intraoperatively. The key to reduction of the posterior malleolus is anatomic reduction and stable fixation of the lateral malleolus. Once this is accomplished, the posterior malleolus can be evaluated and stabilized if necessary. Accurate treatment of the posterior malleolus will help maintain the mortise in an anatomic position and improve stability of the ankle.

References

1. Browner BD, Trafton PG, Green NE, et al. *Skeletal Trauma*. 3rd ed. St. Louis, MO: Elsevier; 2003.
2. Haraguchi N, Haruyama H, Toga H, Kato F. Pathoanatomy of posterior malleolar fractures of the ankle. *J Bone Joint Surg Am*. 2006;88(5):1085-1092.
3. Ebraheim NA, Mekhail AO, Haman SP. External rotation-lateral view of the ankle in the assessment of the posterior malleolus. *Foot Ankle Int*. 1999;20(6):279-283.
4. Raasch WG, Larkin JJ, Draganich LF. Assessment of the posterior malleolus as a restraint to posterior subluxation of the ankle. *J Bone Joint Surg Am*. 1992;74(8):1201-1206.

WHAT IS YOUR POSTOPERATIVE PROTOCOL FOR BIMALLEOLAR ANKLE FRACTURES?

Rajeev Garapati, MD

Postoperative care of the bimalleolar ankle fracture begins in the operating room. Once the fracture is stabilized and the incisions are closed, it is imperative to put a well-padded and molded splint on the patient. I prefer a three-sided plaster splint with the ankle in a neutral position to avoid the development of an equinus contracture. It is also important to elevate the limb in the immediate postoperative period to help decrease the amount of postoperative edema and thus limit the chances of wound complications. The use of ice or cold therapy may also be beneficial to the patient.

The real dilemma and debate regarding postoperative treatment stems from the role of early range of motion (ROM) and weight bearing, and the type of immobilizing devices to use. It has been theorized that early ROM will improve long-term ankle mobility as well as lead to faster rehabilitation and improved articular cartilage nutrition. Similarly, earlier weight bearing could also lead to earlier return of function, not to mention that both earlier ROM and weight bearing make it easier on the patient in the postoperative period. The risk, however, is that both motion and weight bearing increase the forces about the ankle and could lead to fracture displacement.

Numerous different postoperative protocols have been compared in a prospective manner. None of these treatment regimens has led to significantly better results in either the immediate postoperative period or long-term follow-up compared to keeping the patient in a cast for 6 weeks.[1-4] The options include unprotected ROM and weight bearing, protected motion and nonweight bearing, nonweight bearing in a cast, weight bearing in a cast, and active ROM with weight bearing in a CAM boot. Despite the treatment regimen, the long-term ROM of the ankle is similar in all patients. Studies have shown that weight bearing in the early postoperative period has not led to significant fracture displacement or alteration in the final outcome. It also has not led to a more rapid return of function. Early ROM of the ankle, however, does lead to an increased incidence of wound complications and delayed wound healing.[2,4]

Each surgeon must individualize the treatment protocol based on the patient, the fracture, and the fixation achieved.[4] Most patients are discharged home in a splint and a nonweight bearing cast for a period of 2 weeks. At the first follow-up, the wound is evaluated and x-rays are done to evaluate fracture fixation. If everything is stable, further treatment decisions can be made. In young patients with good bone quality and simple fracture patterns in which stable fixation is achieved, it is probably safe to start early ROM and early weight bearing in a CAM boot. In older patients with osteoporosis or complex fracture patterns or less than ideal fixation constructs, it is probably more advisable to place the patient in a nonweight bearing cast for 6 weeks. In highly compliant patients, you can place them in a CAM boot and start early ROM but keep them nonweight bearing until the 6-week mark. It must be noted that the eventual outcome of an ankle fracture is dependent on the position of the mortise at union and not on the initiation of early ROM or weight bearing; thus, I would err on the side of caution in most cases.

At the 6-week mark, most patients can be weight bearing as tolerated and slowly transitioned into regular footwear. A CAM boot or aircast splint can be used for patient comfort but is not routinely necessary. Swelling of the ankle can persist for up to 4 to 6 months postoperatively and so it is advisable for the patient to initially start in lace-up shoes. I will allow them at this time to start nonimpact loading exercises like swimming, elliptical, and exercise bike. I will usually hold them off from running, jumping, and cutting activities until the 3-month mark.

There is some debate as to whether a supervised physical therapy (PT) program is needed in the postoperative period. There is no data in the literature that shows that PT alters short- or long-term outcomes.[5] For this reason, I do not routinely prescribe PT but rather use it on a case-by-case basis. If the patient is not progressing adequately or if he or she is incapable of doing a home exercise program, then a supervised PT program can be useful. It can also be useful in the high functioning athlete who wants to return to sports as quickly as possible.

Most patients with ankle fractures continue to improve for up to 9 months postoperatively. The eventual outcome is good-excellent in 85% to 90% of operatively treated ankle fractures.[5,6] Isolated lateral malleolar fractures do slightly better than bimalleolar or trimalleolar fractures. The most important factor in achieving a good outcome is anatomic reduction of the mortise at union. There are certain fractures that have less favorable results, such as those with significant tibial plafond involvement, anterolateral impaction, injuries to the talar dome, or fractures that are initially widely displaced or dislocated.

One special situation is the diabetic ankle fracture. These patients have an extremely high rate of loss of fixation and infection. They also have a slower than normal healing rate. It is imperative that stable fixation be achieved in the operating room in these patients. Postoperatively, they must be kept nonweight bearing for an extended period of time. My usual protocol for these patients is to keep them in a nonweight bearing cast for a minimum of 6 weeks and sometimes up to 12 weeks. At that time, I will change them to a CAM boot and start some ROM and allow them to be weight bearing as tolerated in the CAM boot for another 6 to 12 weeks. In general, the healing time in diabetics is about twice as long as it is in healthy nondiabetic patients.

In summary, there is no scientific evidence indicating the benefit of early ROM or weight bearing or the institution of PT in the postoperative period. Rather, the surgeon should individualize the program that works best for each patient and each given injury.

What needs to be kept in mind is that patient outcome is more dependent on the anatomic reduction of the fracture and position of the mortise at union than on the postoperative regimen.

References

1. Simanski CJ, Maegele MG, Lefering R, et al. Functional treatment and early weightbearing after an ankle fracture: a prospective study. *J Orthop Trauma*. 2006;20(2):108-114.
2. Lehtonen H, Jarvinen TL, Honkonen S, Nyman M, Vihtonen K, Jarvinen M. Use of a cast compared with a functional ankle brace after operative treatment of an ankle fracture. A prospective, randomized study. *J Bone Joint Surg Am*. 2003;85(2): 205-211.
3. Gul A, Batra S, Mehmood S, Gillham N. Immediate unprotected weight-bearing of operatively treated ankle fractures. *Acta Orthop Belg*. 2007;73(3):360-365.
4. Vioreanu M, Dudeney S, Hurson B, et al. Early mobilization in a removable cast compared with immobilization in a cast after operative treatment of ankle fractures: a prospective randomized study. *Foot Ankle Int*. 2007;28(1):13-19.
5. Bucholz RW, Heckman JD, Court-Brown CM. *Rockwood and Green's Fractures in Adults*. Philadelphia, PA: Lippincott Williams and Wilkins; 2006:2147-2248.
6. Lindsjo U. Operative treatment of ankle fracture-dislocations. a follow-up study of 306/321 consecutive cases. *Clin Orthop*. 1985;199:28-38.

I HAVE AN INSULIN-DEPENDENT 52-YEAR-OLD FEMALE WITH A MINIMALLY DISPLACED BIMALLEOLAR ANKLE FRACTURE. SHOULD I TREAT HER IN A CAST?

Simon Lee, MD

Diabetic patients who present with an orthopedic condition of the foot and ankle require a thorough assessment of their soft tissues and neurovascular status. A history of prior ulcerations or diabetic foot and ankle complications should always raise suspicion of diabetic neuropathy. Clinical examination should include Semmes-Weinstein mono-filament 5.07 nylon testing of bilateral lower extremities. Additional examination should focus on the patient's vascular status. If there is any question, at the minimum a Doppler evaluation of the patient's pulses as well as ankle-brachial index (ABI) or transcutaneous oxygen pressure (T_CPO_2) should be performed to stratify the patient's risk.[1] A vascular consultation should follow as needed. Additionally, laboratory studies should focus on the patient's prior degree of blood glucose control with hemoglobin A1c as well as his or her general nutritional status. Serum albumin levels <3.5 g/dL and total lymphocyte count <1500/mm^3 add to the patient's overall risk factors and prospect of potential complications.

In general, an argument can be made to treat any fracture nonoperatively that is minimally or nondisplaced. In this particular case, however, several factors must be considered. Although a bimalleolar fracture may present with minimal displacement on the latest radiograph, certain factors would compel me toward operative intervention. If the ankle fracture required a reduction or radiographs show a syndesmotic disruption, I would be more apt to pursue operative intervention. These two factors indicate the level of energy imparted to the soft tissues and the degree of soft-tissue stripping and ligamentous instability. I find that these patients do poorly with nonoperative treatment and either continue to displace in a cast or go on to severely delayed malunions. It is obviously helpful to have all radiographs available to make this assessment. Additionally, a patient who presents delayed due to minimal pain or appears to be ambulating on the extremity indicates a level of neuropathy and noncompliance that warrant close follow-up and evaluation as well as more rigid fixation if operative intervention is chosen.[2]

If a patient has significant contraindications to surgery or chooses to be treated conservatively, I place him or her into a well-molded short leg cast or total-contact casting for neuropathic patients as soon as possible. If the patient is still in the acute phase of swelling, the cast will be univalved with a 1-cm strip taken out of the center and then overwrapped with an Ace bandage. The patient is instructed to remain nonweight bearing. Unstable ankle fractures that receive this form of treatment should be followed extremely closely, clinically and radiographically, at weekly intervals until callous formation is seen. As a general rule, a diabetic patient treated in this manner should have all time frames for advancement and healing doubled. For example, they will typically remain nonweight bearing for 6 to 8 weeks, and then advanced to weight bearing as tolerated in a cast for 6 to 8 weeks, and then a cast boot or aircast for an additional 4 to 6 weeks in conjunction with physical therapy. Neuropathic patients may require a Charcot restraint orthotic walker (CROW) after cast removal. If at any time during this treatment the fracture further displaces, operative intervention should be pursued. My threshold to convert to operative treatment is a disruption of the mortise greater than 2 mm.

Operative treatment goals of these patients are the same as for nondiabetics. Most diabetics can undergo open reduction and internal fixation (ORIF) in acute ankle fractures with standard fixation. In a patient who does not have any evidence of neuropathy or osteopenia, standard fixation with a one-third tubular plate on the fibula and cancellous lag screws in the medial malleolus are typically adequate. In my practice, more rigid fixation is mandatory for a patient who is obese, physiologically deconditioned, neuropathic, and/or osteopenic. Depending on the soft-tissue envelope and the degree of soft-tissue tension laterally, I prefer to use a LCD plate or two stacked one-third tubular plates for fixation. I will not hesitate to use multiple syndesmotic screws with three or four cortices fixation if the fibula fixation is poor even without a syndesmotic injury (Figure 38-1). If fixation remains tenuous, increasing to 4.5-mm screws should also be considered. Additionally, for a medial malleolus fracture, I attempt fixation into the posterior or lateral cortices of the tibia for adequate bone purchase. I also use additional medial buttress plating to prevent displacement (Figure 38-2). On occasion, I also encounter extremely unstable fractures, severely osteopenic bone, or a medial soft-tissue envelope that prevents me from immediate medial fixation that requires additional fixation for stability. In these situations, I place a 4- to 5-mm Steinman pin retrograde across the tibiotalar and subtalar joints (see Figure 38-1). These are then cut and tamped in to prevent skin complications and removed even in the office in 3 to 4 months.[3] Postoperatively, the timetable for advancement, as a general rule, is once again doubled. However, I would not hesitate to increase the treatment time frame based on clinical examination. These patients have a high propensity for future foot and ankle complications and should typically be followed on a routine basis even after their fractures are healed.

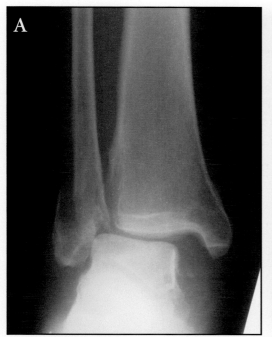
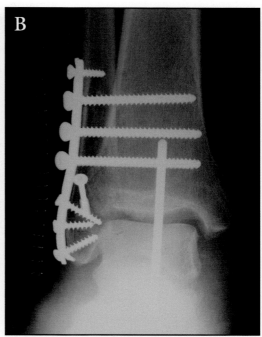

Figure 38-1. (A) An acute displaced distal fibula fracture and deltoid rupture in an insulin-dependent diabetic with mild neuropathy and osteopenia. (B) Postoperative radiographs showing stacked one-third tubular plates, multiple 4.5-mm syndesmotic screw fixation, and a 5-mm Steinman pin placed retrograde across the tibiotalar and subtalar joint for additional stability.

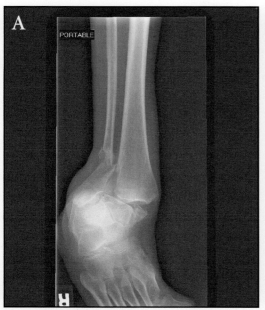
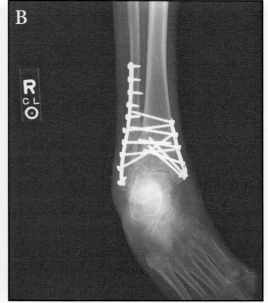

Figure 38-2. (A) A displaced bimalleolar ankle fracture with syndesmotic disruption in an elderly, osteopenic female with insulin-dependent diabetes. (B) Postoperative radiographs showing the use of medial and lateral plating with multiple tibia-fibula trans-osseous cancellous screw fixation to obtain rigid fixation. (Photos courtesy of Christopher Bibbo, DO.)

References

1. Costigan W, Thordarson DB, Debnath UK. Operative management of ankle fractures in patients with diabetes mellitus. *Foot Ankle Int.* 2007;28(1):32-37.
2. Ganesh SP, Pietrobon R, Cecilio WA, Pan D, Lightdale N, Nunly JA. The impact of diabetes on patient outcomes after ankle fracture. *J Bone Joint Surg.* 2005;87(8):1712-1718.
3. Prisk VR, Wukich DK. Ankle fractures in diabetics. *Foot Ankle Clin.* 2006;11(4):849-863.

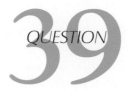

ON WHICH CALCANEAL FRACTURES DO YOU OPERATE?

Robert Vander Griend, MD

From the fracture surgeon's perspective, the calcaneus is a cortical shell surrounded by a fragile soft-tissue envelope with the articular surfaces supported by an internal network of cancellous bone. Axial loading is the common mechanism of injury, resulting in a number of different possible injury patterns and deformities of the calcaneus. This includes injury to the articular surfaces of the posterior, middle, and anterior facets of the subtalar joint and the calcaneo-cuboid joint. The supporting subchondral bone of the subtalar joint is always depressed and often comminuted. The tuberosity may be displaced cephalad, medially into adduction, rotated into varus, shortened along the oblique primary fracture line, or a combination of these deformities. The heel is widened as the lateral wall and occasionally medial wall are displaced. In addition, the surrounding soft tissues are damaged by the initial trauma, displacement of bony fragments, and the resultant swelling.

Controversy exists as to how much deformity can be accepted. Regardless, it is clear that injury and residual incongruity of the articular surfaces predisposes to loss of motion and post-traumatic arthritis. The depression of the central calcaneus affects the subtalar joint, but also enables the talar body to settle into dorsiflexion, compromising the function of the ankle. Persistent widening of the lateral wall often results in impingement and peroneal tendon problems. These problems plus the deformities of the heel as noted above can result in chronic pain and swelling, gait disturbances, shoe wear problems, and functional and vocational limitations.

As a result, the goals in treating these displaced intra-articular fractures are to restore the articular surfaces and supporting bone using fixation with sufficient stability to maintain this alignment and permit early motion of the injured joints. Numerous studies have shown that these goals can be achieved, but the complication rates are high primarily due to compromised soft tissues and patient comorbidities.[1] Despite the complication rates, it is generally believed that open reduction and internal fixation (ORIF) of these fractures gives better results than nonoperative treatment. However, in this era of evidence-based medicine, this has been difficult to prove.

Buckley,[2] in a series of studies resulting from a prospective, randomized, controlled multicenter trial on operative compared with nonoperative treatment of displaced intra-articular calcaneus fractures, found that some subgroups of patients had better outcomes after surgical treatment. Better outcomes were noted in females, younger patients, and patients who did not have to return to heavy workloads and/or were not receiving workers compensation. Patients with lower classification grades (ie, less comminution), anatomic reduction of the posterior facet or a step off of <2 mm, and restoration of Bohler's angle also had better outcomes. Unfortunately, the remaining patients (males, overweight, higher degrees of comminution, heavy workload, work-related) did not do well with nonoperative treatment either. The question therefore remains: Which fractures in which patients should be treated with ORIF?

My indications for ORIF in these fractures include:

* Two- or three-part fractures of the posterior facet (Sanders Type II or III) with depression of the articular surfaces more than 2 mm to 3 mm on computed tomography (CT) scan
* Displacement of the lateral wall of the calcaneus beyond the lateral edge of the fibula (patients may have symptomatic impingement with less displacement but they are all symptomatic with this much displacement)
* Displacement of the tuberosity resulting in compromise of the soft tissues or a hindfoot deformity that will cause problems with shoe wear and walking, especially a varus and/or adduction malunion of the heel
* Soft tissues suitable for surgical treatment
* Patient suitable for surgical treatment (A detailed and thorough informed consent is essential. In terms of patient comorbidities, diabetes, obesity, peripheral vascular disease, and smoking seem to be particularly important risk factors.)

Some of these fractures are amenable to percutaneous reduction and fixation techniques. If the articular surfaces are restored and the surrounding bone is realigned, the results of these techniques seem comparable to those with formal open reduction utilizing an extensile exposure. However, more study of these minimally invasive options is needed. There also may be a role for percutaneous techniques to improve the alignment of the heel when soft tissue compromises and patient factors preclude an open reduction.

The highly comminuted calcaneus fracture (Sanders IV) is probably destined to need a subtalar fusion. The unresolved question is whether to do this as a primary procedure (when soft tissue permits) or as a delayed reconstruction.

Finally, it should be noted that surgeon experience is important in treating these injuries. These are difficult fractures not well-suited for the occasional fracture surgeon. The surrounding soft tissues are unforgiving and resulting problems difficult to salvage. Open internal fixation (ie, without reduction) exposes patients to all the risks of operative treatment but few of the benefits. Fractures of the calcaneus are seldom emergencies, so there is ample time for a thorough evaluation, observation of the soft tissues, and transfer of the patient, if needed.

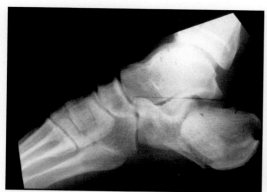

Figure 39-1A. Lateral radiograph: Intra-articular fracture of the calcaneous.

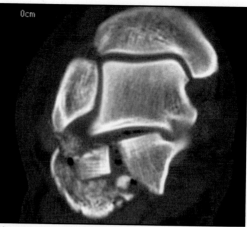

Figure 39-1B. Coronal CT scan shows displacement of the posterior facet and the lateral wall of the calcaneous with subfibular impingement.

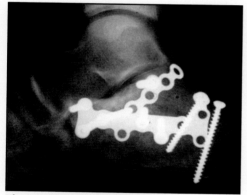

Figure 39-1C. Postoperative radiograph after open reduction and internal fixation.

References

1. Sanders R. Displaced intra-articular fractures of the calcaneus. *J Bone Joint Surg Am.* 2000;82:225-250.
2. Buckley R, Tough S, McCormack R, Pate G, Leighton R, Petrie D, Galpin R. Operative compared with nonoperative treatment of displaced intra-articular calcaneal fractures. *J Bone Joint Surg Am.* 84:1733-1744.

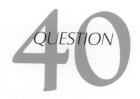

THERE IS A PATIENT IN THE ER WITH A DISPLACED TALAR NECK FRACTURE. WHAT IS THE TECHNIQUE FOR FIXATION?

Armen S. Kelikian, MD

When evaluating a fracture of the talus, my preference for radiographs is an anterior-posterior (AP), lateral, and internal and external rotation views of the foot. A Canale view is paramount. This is performed with the ankle in plantar flexion, the foot is pronated about 15 degrees, while the x-ray beam is angled cephalad 75 degrees from the floor. This pronated oblique view of the midfoot can detect any angular deformity of the talar head and neck relative to the body as well as any displacement. A varus deformity is most common in Type II fractures. A computed tomography (CT) scan is useful to detect subtle changes to differentiate between a Type I and Type II fracture, neck comminution, or body involvement, which is usually in the sagittal plane.[1]

Talar neck fractures are classified by the Canale-Kelly system: Type I—undisplaced neck fracture, Type II—displacement seen at the subtalar joint (Figure 40-1), Type III—displacement at the subtalar and ankle joint, and Type IV—extrusion from the ankle mortise and talonavicular joint. The incidence of avascular necrosis is 0%, 50%, 90%, and 100% in the four corresponding fracture types. The mortise ankle view at 8 weeks will show subchondral lucency under the talar dome, which denotes vascular exchange in the nonweight bearing limb. This is referred to as positive Hawkins's sign (Figure 40-2). There is a 5% false-positive reading in adults and it is less reliable in the pediatric population. Some literature purports that there is a lower rate of AVN in cases treated with immediate open reduction and internal fixation (ORIF) (ie, within 6 to 8 hours), but two recent studies refute this.[2]

While closed reduction of displaced talus fractures can be attempted, anatomic reduction is difficult to both achieve and assess radiographically. On the lateral side, as little as 3 degrees of varus tilt will result in significant loss of subtalar joint. Taking this into account, you should carefully scrutinize any attempt at indirect reduction techniques. I use a tenaculum to grasp the talar head and place it on the body akin to a scoop of ice cream on a cone (Figure 40-3).

Figure 40-1. Displaced Type II talar neck fracture.

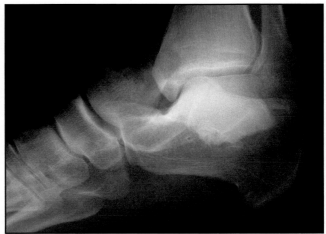

Figure 40-2. Hawkin's sign at 8 weeks postoperative shows lucency (+ sign) laterally but not in the medial talar dome.

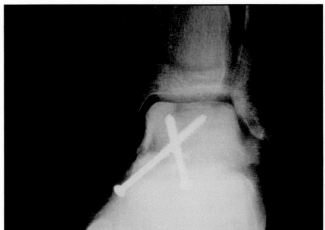

Figure 40-3. Indirect reduction using a large tenaculum.

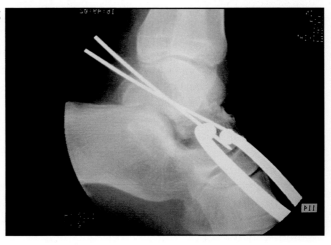

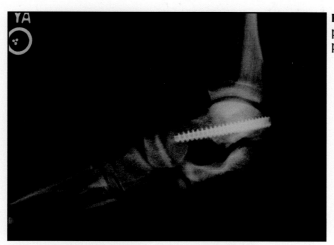

Figure 40-4. Posterior-anterior compression with a tapered variable pitch cannulated 7/6-mm screw.

Type II fractures can be treated open via a lateral sinus tarsi approach and if necessary a supplemental medial ankle approach. The former visualizes the subtalar joint for incongruity while the latter allows inspection of the ankle articulation. Be careful not to damage the deep deltoid ligament since it may be the only viable vessel left in Type II fractures. I prefer a 45-degree positioning with the leg on a padded build up. The sinus tarsus is exposed and the fracture is accessed. If the reduction is not anatomic, I proceed to the lateral approach first. The sinus tarsi are exposed via a linear incision that starts at the tip of the fibula and proceeds distally in line with the fourth metatarsal. The peroneal tendons are identified and retracted with a Penrose drain. For body fractures, a medial malleolar osteotomy is safer for exposure unless there is an associated medial malleolus fracture (20%). The screw holes are predrilled and the malleolus is hinged on the deltoid ligament. This allows excellent exposure of the talar body as well as neck.

Intraoperative traction using a standard femoral distractor medially with a pin in the calcaneous and tibia can facilitate the reduction. K-wires may also assist in the reduction and can be used as a joystick to maneuver the neck and head fragment. Comminution is usually medial and dorsal and on occasion will require bone grafting as well as medial plating.

Various options are available in the armamentarium for internal fixation. Posterior to anterior screw fixation (6.5-mm to 7.3-mm cannulated lag screws) via a posterolateral percutaneous approach gives fixation perpendicular to the fracture line (Figure 40-4). Biomechanically, it is superior to two retrograde crossed screws (Figure 40-5).

Depending on the location of the fracture line, one of these screws may have a small osseous bridge. Be aware in cases of medial comminution to avoid excess compression. When the fracture is close to the talar head's reticular surface, a headless screw is preferable. Recently, in cases of medial comminution, mini-fragment (2.7 mm) locked plates have been used medially as well as laterally to maintain the length of either respective side (Figure 40-6).

I generally use a bulky cotton Jones compression dressing with a U splint for 2 weeks. After this time, the sutures are removed and a short leg cast is applied and patient is nonweight bearing for an additional 3 weeks. The cast is then removed and replaced with a removable prefabricated posterior splint in a neutral position. Isometric and eccentric

Figure 40-5. ORIF with two retrograde screws.

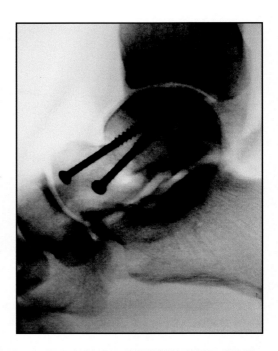

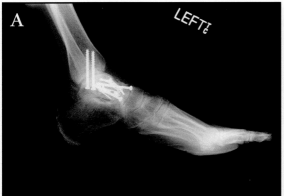

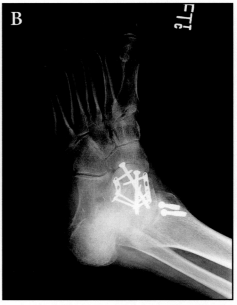

Figure 40-6. (A) Type II talar neck fracture treated with two retrograde screws and two mini-fragmentation plates because of medial comminution. (B) Canale view.

muscle strengthening exercises are begun at this time for invertors/evertors as well as dorsi and plantar flexors. Don't forget to check for a positive Hawkins' sign at 6 to 8 weeks. Weight bearing is begun at the time of fracture union, which is about 3 months postoperatively.

Long-term problems and complications should be discussed with the patient early in treatment. These include avascular necrosis, arthritis, malunion, nonunion, as well as abnormal kinematics and joint stiffness. Late reconstructive surgery is not uncommon.

References

1. Kelikian AS. Fractures of the talus. In: *Operative Treatment of the Foot and Ankle*. Stamford, CT: Appleton & Lange; 1999:496-516.
2. Juliano PJ, Dabbah M, Harris TG. Talar neck fractures. *Foot Ankle Clin*. 2004;9(4):723-736.

WHICH METATARSAL FRACTURES NEED SURGERY?

Johnny L. Lin, MD

Metatarsal fractures are the most common fracture of the foot. Mechanism of injury is usually twisting of the foot, followed by falls and direct blows. High-energy injuries (ie, motor vehicle collisions) should heighten one's suspicion of associated Lisfranc injuries. Metatarsal fractures resulting from gun shot wounds (GSW) should be treated as open fractures.

Examination reveals swelling over the dorsum of the foot with pain to direct palpation over the fractured metatarsals. The "pathway" of the injury should be determined, with particular attention given to joints bordering the metatarsal fractures (Figure 41-1). Spontaneous reduction may have occurred in a bordering joint despite significant ligamentous injury. Neurovascular exam and testing for compartment syndrome should be carried out, including palpation, passive stretching of compartments, and noting pain out of proportion. Compartment pressure readings are not routinely obtained. Finally, the metatarsal heads should be palpated for plantar prominence or absence with the foot and ankle simulating the stance phase of gait.

Radiographic examination includes three views of the foot. Acute weight bearing or stress views of the foot are usually not possible without sedation or local anesthetic. In the acute setting, local anesthetic is not recommended because it impairs serial neurologic examination. If additional injuries are suspected, a computed tomography (CT) scan can also be obtained.

Central metatarsal fractures are frequently underestimated due to their benign appearance. As a result, poor outcomes are common (40% to 60%). Unfortunately, there are few quality studies to guide treatment. Widely accepted thresholds for closed reduction and/or surgical fixation are shortening greater than 4 mm to 5 mm and sagittal plane angulation greater than 10 degrees. These parameters seem to correlate with the development of metatarsalgia, which is the most common reason for a poor result. I additionally consider a clinically prominent or absent metatarsal head plantarly as an indication for interven-

Figure 41-1. The "pathway" of the injury for a second metatarsal shaft fracture that was the result of a Lisfranc equivalent injury with disruption of the first metatarsal-cuneiform joint.

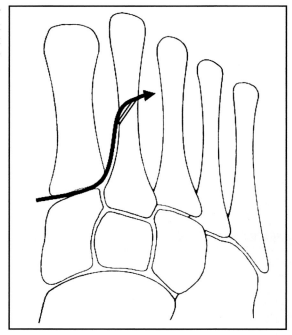

tion, regardless of radiographic appearance. Coronal angulation does not appear to have long-term consequences. If nonsurgical treatment is instituted, healing should occur in 6 weeks. Immediate weight bearing is allowed for isolated fractures. Those with multiple metatarsal fractures are kept nonweight bearing for 4 weeks in a postoperative shoe. Surgical fixation is preferred if an adequate reduction cannot be obtained or maintained. There are no comparative studies to guide choice of implant or technique. When possible, I prefer closed reduction and longitudinal pinning of the metatarsal with a 2.0-mm k-wire to preserve the soft-tissue envelope. Weight bearing and k-wire removal occur at 6 weeks. Alternative forms of fixation include mini-fragment plates or transverse pinning of the distal and proximal fragment to a bordering metatarsal. I use these techniques only when longitudinal k-wires fail to maintain an adequate reduction.

Fifth metatarsal fractures can be classified and treated according to location and chronicity. There are three types of proximal fractures (Figure 41-2). Type I (pseudo-Jones fracture) injuries are treated weight bearing as tolerated with a postoperative shoe. Union rate at 4 to 6 weeks is >90%. Type II injuries (Jones fracture) are treated with a nonweight bearing short-leg cast for 6 to 8 weeks. The union rate is 70% to 90%, but healing can take up to 21 weeks. Early open reduction and internal fixation (ORIF) can be considered in the athlete to quicken recovery time. Type of fixation is surgeon preference. I prefer a partially threaded cannulated system using the largest implant accommodated by the diaphysis, but use at least a 4.5-mm screw (Figure 41-3). Union rate is 90% to 100% at 6 to 8 weeks. Type III injuries occur in the diaphysis and may be the result of a stress fracture. If acute, they can be treated in the same manner as a Type II fracture. Sclerosis and narrowing of the canal indicate a chronic condition. I prefer to fix these in the same manner as described above. Union rate is 90% to 100% at 8 to 10 weeks.

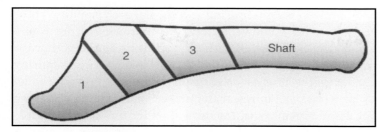

Figure 41-2. Proximal fifth metatarsal fracture classification by location. (© 1995 American Academy of Orthopaedic Surgeons. Reprinted from the *Journal of the American Academy of Orthopaedic Surgeons*, Volume 3(2), pp. 110-114 with permission.)

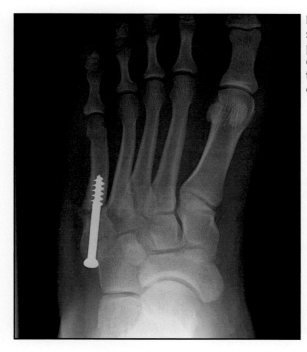

Figure 41-3A. AP radiograph of a 6.5 mm short-thread solid stainless steel screw placed after drilling with the 4.5 mm cannulated system. Notice all the screw threads across the fracture site and the central position.

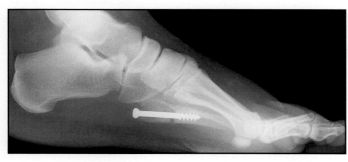

Figure 41-3B. Lateral radiograph verifying central position of the screw with all threads crossing the fracture site.

The first metatarsal has a vital role in weight bearing and medial arch stability. These fractures are treated nonsurgically with a nonweight bearing short-leg cast for 6 to 8 weeks only if nondisplaced and nonangulated. Any displacement or angulation at the time of injury or during nonsurgical treatment signifies an unstable fracture requiring surgical fixation. Surgical implant and technique are surgeon preference. I prefer a small fragment T-plate for shaft or proximal metaphyseal fractures. Small fragment locking plates can also be helpful. For distal metaphyseal fractures, I prefer multiple 2.0-mm k-wires. Articular involvement with displacement >1 mm should be fixed using absorbable pins or headless screws.

Despite the common occurrence of these fractures, they are commonly ignored or reflexively treated nonoperatively. Avoiding significant disability requires vigilance in ruling out more severe injuries and paying close attention to the metatarsal's role in weight bearing. Although few require surgery, failure to recognize and treat these fractures appropriately results in a high percentage of patients with long-term disability.

References

1. Armagan OE, Shereff MJ. Injuries to the toes and metatarsals. *Orthop Clin North Am.* 2001;32(1):1-10.
2. Early JS. Fractures and dislocations of the midfoot and forefoot. In: Bucholz RW, Heckman JD, eds. *Rockwood and Green's: Fractures in Adults.* 5th ed. Philadelphia, PA: Lippincott, Williams and Wilkins; 2002.
3. Holmes GB. Gunshot wounds of the foot. *Clin Orthop.* 2003;(408):86-91.
4. Petrisor BA, Ekrol I, Court-Brown C. The epidemiology of metatarsal fractures. *Foot Ankle Int.* 2006;27(3):172-174.
5. Sanchez Alepuz E, Vicent Carsi V, Alcantara P, Llabres AJ. Fractures of the central metatarsal. *Foot Ankle Int.* 11996;7(4):200-203.

DO YOU EVER BONE GRAFT ACUTE FRACTURES?

Dave Dean, DO
Bruce H. Ziran, MD

Historically, autograft has been the standard of care for bone defects. Unfortunately, it carries significant morbidity and has limited supply. As a result, grafting of fractures has been done on a delayed basis because of concerns regarding infection, limited supply, and success rates. Improved surgical technique including debridement and microvascular free flaps have reduced the infection risk and allow the consideration for acute bone grafting. Kesemenli et al[1] showed union in 19/20 open tibia fractures with a 5% infection rate, which were treated with stabilization and bone grafting within 24 hours of injury.

Grafts function as osteoconductive, osteoinductive, or osteosupportive agents. An osteoconductive graft provides a scaffold for osteoprogenitor cells to attach and form new bone. Osteoconductive options include allograft, ceramics, and the newer resorbable bone cements. Similar to osteoconductive options are osteosupportive products. The osteosupportive grafts are essentially osteoconductive grafts whose use should be restricted to subarticular applications, such as contained defects under periarticular reconstructions. We typically use calcium phosphate in settings that require mechanical support, as it has been shown to be superior to cancellous graft.[2] We reserve calcium sulfate for use as a resorbable antibiotic depot because it has low compressive strength and resorbs quickly—in about 6 weeks. Also, calcium sulfate has an osmotic effect that can result in drainage and complications. As such, the ceramic products should not be used for femoral neck fractures or for diaphyseal or metaphyseal defects because they will only serve to block appropriate biologic healing at the fracture site. Osteoinductive grafts promote cellular formation of bone and usually work via protein signaling. Osteoinductive options include autograft, demineralized bone matrix (DBM), and the very potent bone morphogenetic proteins (BMP). For contained metaphyseal defects, DBM has been shown to be comparable to autograft,[4] and for open tibial fractures, BMP has been shown to be superior to no graft use.[5] Most DBM studies, however, are level III or IV studies and lack appropriate studies that demonstrate their true clinical and economic efficiency.

The choice to use one over the other has to take into account the severity of injury and medical comorbidities that would increase the likelihood of developing a delayed union or nonunion, as well as the cost and effectiveness of the graft material chosen. Our choice to acutely bone graft fractures is based on the severity and location of the injury. In the acute closed diaphyseal fracture, grafting is rarely if ever needed. Even in highly comminuted closed fractures, there is a good chance of healing if proper surgical technique is used.

In closed metaphyseal and periarticular fractures, we prefer to use DBM or a calcium phosphate cement. One of the authors has shown favorable success rates of DBM in metaphyseal fractures.[4] Calcium phosphate cements can be easily injected into defects, but care must be taken to avoid any extravasation through articular cracks into the joint. Calcium phosphate has been shown to have a higher compressive strength than cancellous bone,[2] and is absorbed much slower than calcium sulfate. If the metaphyseal fracture is open, we would ensure a clean tissue bed, but use DBM preferentially because if an infection occurs, it would be easier to remove than well-interdigitated calcium cement. It is important to understand that calcium phosphate cements are osteoconductive and osteosupportive only. They provide mechanical support until replaced by creeping substitution and are not bone union accelerators. In contrast, DBM grafts are both inductive agents as well as conductive, but their mechanical support is not as good as cements.

In the diaphyseal location, there is little evidence to support acute grafting of closed fracture, but there is Level I evidence for the use of BMP[2] in severe open fractures. Considering that many patients with such severe fractures have host factors that predispose them to nonunion (nutrition, nicotine, compliance, etc), and are also uninsured, they are paradoxically the best suited for use of such effective agents. We feel that use of BMP in this setting gives the best chance of success and saves pelvic autograft for later use should it be necessary. There is no role yet for use of cements in diaphyseal fractures.

In general, grafting of open fracture acutely remains controversial. Yet, with modern debridement techniques it may be possible to do so safely. Irrespective of the location, it is essential to do so with a clean tissue bed. Frequently, this involves more than one debridement and the use of antibiotic laden beads. Our preference is to place the graft at the time of definitive closure. In some low grade fractures with a little bone loss (eg, Grade II, open both bone fracture), one may consider using DBM as an inductive and conductive graft acutely.

When considering a graft option, consider the location and function of the graft. Autograft remains the gold standard but carries a known morbidity. DBM, allograft, and bone cements are best suited for contained defects or support of articular segments. In diaphyseal and meta-diaphyseal locations, osteoinduction and osteogenesis is required so cements are less suited for this role and DBM, allograft, and BMP are better options (Figures 42-1 through 42-3).

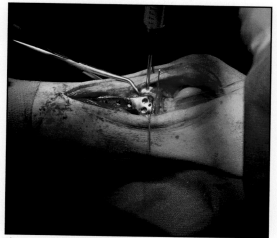

Figure 42-1. The injection of calcium phosphate cement into a tibial plateau defect.

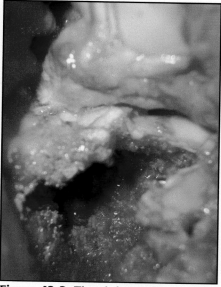

Figure 42-2. The defect below a tibial plateau.

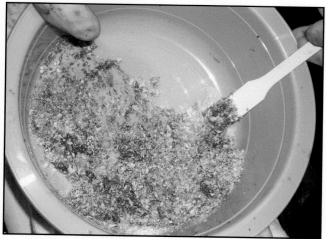

Figure 42-3. Mixture of DBM with crushed cancellous allograft.

References

1. Kesemenli C, et al. Early prophylactic autogenous bone grafting in type III open tibial fractures. *Acta Orthop Belg.* 2004;70:327-331.
2. Trenholm A, et al. Comparative fixation of tibial plateau fractures using α-BSM, a calcium phosphate cement, versus cancellous bone graft. *J Orthop Trauma.* 2005;19:698-702.
3. Kelly C, Wilkins R, Gitelis S, Hartjen C, Watson JT, Kim P. The use of a surgical grade calcium sulfate as a bone graft substitute. *Clin Orthop.* 2001;382:42-50.
4. Cheung S, Westerheide K, Ziran B. Efficacy of contained metaphyseal and periarticular defects treated with two different demineralized bone matrix allografts. *Int Orthop.* 2003;27:56-59.
5. Govender S, Csimma C, Genant H, Opran A. Recombinant human bone morphogenetic protein-2 for treatment of open tibial fractures. *J Bone Joint Surg,* 2002;84:2123-2134.

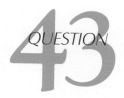

I HAVE A 34-YEAR-OLD MALE WITH A NONUNION OF A PLATED MIDSHAFT TIBIA FRACTURE. HOW DO YOU APPROACH THIS PROBLEM?

Stuart M. Gold, MD

When I am referred a nonunion for consultation and treatment, I try to determine if I am dealing with a biologic or a mechanical problem. In many cases, this can be determined by the x-ray alone; however, obtaining an accurate history from the onset of the injury always provides critical information.

The significant questions I ask include mechanism of injury (high or low energy); open or closed fracture; and whether significant soft-tissue, vascular, or neurologic injury occurred. Additionally, I inquire about the initial treatment management the patient underwent, ie, splinting versus temporary external fixation, the length of time the temporary fixation was in place, and if there were any pin track issues. I determine if there were any wound issues or wound drainage at any time, including the initial or later phases of treatment, as well as the development of any deformity during the treatment period. Finally, the length of time from the initial injury to presentation and the number and types of surgeries as well as possible bone grafts and/or types of bone grafting material are important queries.

Following all of these critical history questions, I carry out a thorough physical examination to assess deformity, ie, angulation, shortening, malrotation, and most importantly, the mechanical axis of the limb and the stiffness of the nonunion. I then carefully determine the status of the soft-tissue envelope, most notably around the nonunion as well as proximal and distal to the nonunion, to determine if it will tolerate violation with an extensive open surgery. The function of both the knee and the foot also need to be carefully assessed.

Radiographs are then reviewed to help assess the biology for any evidence of callus or any evidence of infection or for bone that clearly does not have healing potential.

Comparison films from the contralateral limb are helpful, as are long mechanical axis films from the hip to the ankle. If a deformity is present, the specifics such as bone loss, shortening, or whether a gap is present need to be assessed. Additionally, overall shortening or angulation or rotational deformity needs to be determined to see if they can all be corrected at the time of the definitive treatment of the nonunion.

Other forms of testing can be helpful, but are rarely definitive with respect to determining if an infection is present. These include laboratory tests such as white blood cell counts, ESR, C-reactive protein, as well as more invasive tests such as technetium bone scans, Indium-111 scans, and magnetic resonance imaging (MRI) scans; however, it is my opinion that infection is usually best determined by history, physical examination, and deep cultures; the other methods are only occasionally helpful.

In this case with a 34-year-old male with a nonunion of plate at the midshaft tibia, the key issue is to determine if it is a biologic or mechanical problem. My specific treatment plan is directly related to the issues of infection as well as the status of the soft-tissue envelope surrounding the nonunion. If this is purely a mechanical problem, there is no sign of infection, but there is good healing potential, my choice of refixation will then depend on the soft-tissue envelope. During open plate removal, a gram stain, deep cultures, and a frozen section are taken, which provide me with the definitive answer with respect to infection.

Assuming no infection, my preferred approach is for an intramedullary, reamed nail locked at both ends, correcting any mechanical axis deformities at the time of nailing. Additionally, I place a bone graft either using an autogenous cancellous iliac crest or a combination of a demineralized bone matrix or cancellous chips with marrow aspirate. I believe that opening the nonunion site to remove the plate affects the local biology enough to warrant bone grafting, even in the setting of a hypertrophic nonunion. If a nail, for whatever reason, was not feasible, then replating with a longer plate would be a second option; again, assuring mechanical axis is aligned as well as providing a graft as noted above.

If found to be an infected nonunion, my approach is different in that the hardware needs to be removed, followed by a resection of all the necrotic or infected bone, assuring that healthy bone with healing potential is evident on both sides of the gap. My treatment then depends on the virulence of the organism and the residual bone defect after debridement. If I had a gap of less than 3 cm, I place an antibiotic nail for 6 to 12 weeks, to be followed by an exchange nail and bone grafting using the grafting options as noted above. If the gap was greater than 3 cm and since I am comfortable with bone transports, I proceed with a circular frame and bone transport. The gap would be filled with antibiotic impregnated cement, a combination of vancomycin and tobramycin in the appropriate ratio for 6 to 8 weeks then followed by removal of the antibiotic impregnated beads and then start of the bone transport. At that point, I decide if the docking site requires a bone graft prior to its completion of docking.

In conclusion, the key reasons I have used a circular fixator for nonunions of the tibia include infected gaps greater than 3 cm, nonunions associated with shortening, and significant deformities with poor soft-tissue envelopes. As many circular fixators as I apply, I still nail and plate a significantly greater number of fractures and non/malunions per year.

Suggested Reading

Gold SM, Wasserman R. Preliminary results of tibial bone transports with pulsed low intensity ultrasound (exogen). *J Ortho Trauma*. 2005;19:10-16.

Mckee MD, Schemitsch EH, Waddell JP. The use of an antibiotic-impregnated osteoconductive, bioabsorbable bone substitute in the treatment of infected long bone defects. Early results of a prospective trial. *J Ortho Trauma*. 2002;16:622-627.

Stoffel K, Dieter U, Stachowiak G, Gachter A, Kuster MS. Biomechanical testing of the LCP: how can stability in locked internal fixation be controlled? *Injury*. 2003;34(supp 2):B11-B19.

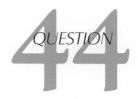

How Do I Treat a Child With a Twisted Ankle and Normal X-Rays?

Monica Kogan, MD

Ankle injuries in children are common. They may occur during a sporting event or while running around at recess. Children will present with swelling, pain, and at times inability to bear weight. The diagnosis can vary from an ankle fracture to an ankle sprain, and it can often be difficult to differentiate between the two in a skeletally immature patient.

A child who presents to the office or emergency department with a history of pain and swelling after a trauma most likely has some pathology present. A full history and physical examination should be performed. Both the bony anatomy as well as the ligamentous anatomy should be palpated. This should include the anterior, posterior, and calcaneofibular ligaments, the deltoid ligaments, and the syndesmosis. The distal tibia, medial and lateral malleolus, as well as the area of the physis on the tibia and fibula should all be palpated. Pain with active or passive range of motion should be noted and neurovascular status should be assessed.

The Ottawa Rules are guidelines for the necessity of radiographs in the acute setting.[1] These guidelines were developed for the adult population; in the skeletally immature patient, I take a different approach. When a child presents with the above symptoms, even if he or she is an adolescent and may look like an adult, radiographs are obtained. These include anterior-posterior (AP), lateral, and mortise views evaluating for any signs of fracture, displacement, or disruption of the mortise.

Often the radiographs will not show any obvious abnormalities and the patient is diagnosed with an ankle sprain. Current literature supports functional treatment for ankle sprains in adults, which includes three phases.[2] The first phase includes protection, rest, ice, compression, and elevation. During this phase, the patient is encouraged to use crutches until able to bear weight without discomfort, after which he or she progresses to phases two and three; this may take 2 to 3 days. Phases two and three consist of progressive stretching followed by strengthening and conditioning.

The mentioned protocol, however, is described for adults. When faced with this clinical situation in a child, I place the patient in a below-the-knee weight bearing cast for a period of 4 weeks. After the cast is removed, physical therapy is begun, which includes stretching, strengthening and proprioception.

My approach is conservative for many reasons. First of all, because the physis is still open, the patient may have a Salter-Harris I fracture of the tibia or fibula that may not be obvious on the radiographs and needs to be protected. Salter-Harris I fractures are through the physis and not always easily identified on the radiographs. Often the only radiographic finding is on follow-up films, where callus may be visible.

Secondly, children are not just "smaller adults." Their attitude toward slowing down their activity is completely different. As soon as pediatric patients begin to feel better, they typically are back to their regular activity level. More often than not, skeletally immature patients want to get back to performing the sport they love or get back to recess as soon as possible, even if the sprain/injury is not completely healed. This can be as soon as 1 to 2 weeks, which is too early to be returning to their preinjury level of play, as the injury is still healing. By immobilizing the ankle, the injury has time to adequately heal and the patients are not tempted by their friends/coaches to get back to participating in their desired activities before their ankles are ready.

I have seen numerous patients who have sustained ankle injuries that were diagnosed as sprains and who were treated like "little adults." They were given crutches, an aircast, and were told to begin walking on it when the ankle felt better. The injuries never had a chance to heal because the patients began running on them before the ankles were ready for the stress. It is for this reason that skeletally immature patients need to be immobilized. This can be in a cast, or if the patient will be compliant, a CAM walker.

The approach to a skeletally immature patient with a history of a twisted ankle and normal x-ray films should be treated very conservatively and should not be treated in the same fashion as treating an adult patient with similar symptoms. In doing so, the injury, either ligamentous or bony, will have time to heal and may prevent any future symptoms from occurring secondary to having an inadequately healed injury.

References

1. Chorley JN, Hergenroeder AC. Management of ankle sprains. *Pediatric Annals. 1997*;26(1):56-66.
2. Trevino SG, Davis P, Hecht PJ. Management of acute and chronic lateral ligament injuries of the ankle. *Orthop Clin of North Am.* 1994;25(1):1-15.

How Do You Assess Compartment Syndrome of the Foot?

Johnny L. Lin, MD

Compartment syndrome of the foot is a frequently overlooked diagnosis. The pathophysiology of the condition is identical to leg compartment syndrome (which is more common and will not be covered in this chapter). The most common etiology is trauma, including metatarsal fractures, Lisfranc fractures/dislocations, calcaneus fractures, and crush injuries. Chronic sequelae of foot compartment syndrome include claw toes, cavus deformity, and sensory neuropathy. The exact incidence of this condition is unknown because it is rare and frequently missed. In a large retrospective study, 5% of calcaneus fractures had late clawing of the toes, consistent with a missed compartment syndrome. From this data, it is estimated that 10% of calcaneus fractures have a clinically apparent compartment syndrome because approximately 50% of compartment syndromes will develop clawing.[1] Nontraumatic compartment syndrome of the foot from a slow bleed into a confined foot compartment can also occur, but is extremely rare.

The diagnosis of a compartment syndrome of the foot is similar to the diagnosis in the leg. One must maintain a high clinical suspicion in cases of high-energy trauma, especially in the setting of a crush injury. The major complaint is inconsolable pain, except in late cases. Common findings are pain from passive extension of the toes and decreased two-point discrimination (>5 mm to 7 mm). Motor loss, delayed capillary refill, and loss of palpable pulses are uncommon.[2] I prefer Doppler examination when pulses are non-palpable due to swelling.

Measurement of compartment pressures can also be carried out to verify the diagnosis. This requires a working knowledge of the location and number of compartments in the foot. The most commonly accepted description of the compartments of the foot is the nine-compartment model.[3] There are three compartments (lateral, medial, and superficial) that run the length of the foot. Additionally, there are four separate compartments for each of the interossei, one for the adductor hallucis, and a calcaneal compartment

Table 45-1

Contents of the Compartments of the Foot

Compartment	Important Structures
Medial	• Abductor hallucis • Flexor hallucis
Lateral	• Abductor digiti quinti • Flexor digiti minimi
Superficial	• Flexor digitorum brevis • Lumbricals[4] • Flexor digitorum longus tendons • +/- Medial plantar nerve, artery, and vein
Interosseus[4]	• Plantar and dorsal interossei
Adductor	• Adductor hallucis
Calcaneal	• Quadratus plantae • Tibial nerve, artery, and vein • Lateral plantar nerve, artery, and vein • +/- Medial plantar nerve, artery, and vein

(or deep hindfoot compartment). The contents of each of these compartments are listed in Table 45-1. There are several different methods to measure pressures, but I prefer to use a stic device (Stryker, Kalamazoo, MI) because of its portability and ease of use. In order to measure the pressure in the interosseous compartment, the needle is introduced dorsally between the metatarsals, approximately 1 cm deep. The adductor compartment is measured by advancing the needle an additional 3 cm to 4 cm within the first interosseus compartment. The lateral compartment is measured by introducing the needle just inferior to the base of the fifth metatarsal. The medial compartment is measured approximately 4 cm inferior to the medial malleolus over the abductor hallucis. Advancement of the needle an additional 3 cm to 4 cm allows measurement of the calcaneal compartment. Of note, the calcaneal compartment has a direct communication with the deep posterior compartment of the leg, making it susceptible to the transfer of elevated pressures. The superficial compartment can be entered by placing the needle between the inferior edge of the abductor hallucis and the plantar fascia and advancing 3 cm to 4 cm. Absolute pressures >30 mm Hg and values within 10 to 30 mm Hg of the diastolic pressure have been used as criteria for surgical.[4,5]

If surgical release is indicated, it should be done ideally within the first 8 hours. Delayed release (12 to 24 hours) should be avoided due to the high incidence of infection. There are several techniques described for compartment release. I prefer a combined dorsal and medial approach. The dorsal approach consists of two longitudinal incisions, one just medial to the second metatarsal and one just lateral to the fourth metatarsal. All interosseous compartments can be released using these two incisions. The adductor compartment is released through the floor of the first web space (Figure 45-1). The remaining compartments are released through a medial incision made parallel to the plantar surface

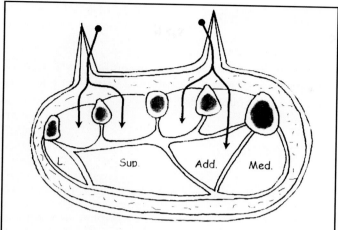

Figure 45-1. Dorsal incisions allow release of interosseous compartments and adductor compartment. (Copyright © 2008 by the American Orthopaedic Foot and Ankle Society, Inc., originally published in *Foot & Ankle Int.* 2003;24(2):180-187 and reproduced here with permission.)

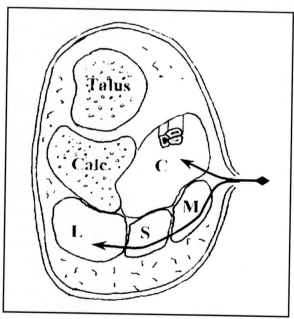

Figure 45-2. Medial incision allows release of the medial (M), calcaneal (C), superficial (S), and lateral compartment (L). (Copyright © 2008 by the American Orthopaedic Foot and Ankle Society, Inc., originally published in *Foot & Ankle Int.* 2003;24(2):180-187 and reproduced here with permission.)

of the foot, starting approximately 4 cm anterior to the posterior heel and 3 cm superior to the plantar surface of the foot. The medial compartment is entered first, followed by superior retraction of the muscle belly of the abductor hallucis in order to gain access to the deep fascia. By incising the deep fascia, the calcaneal compartment is released. Care must be taken to avoid the lateral plantar nerve during this release. The superficial compartment is entered by subcutaneous dissection just below the abductor hallucis until the fascia of the superficial compartment is identified and incised. Plantar retraction of the flexor digitorum brevis within the superficial compartment and dissection laterally reveals the medial wall of the lateral compartment, which can then be released through the superficial compartment (Figure 45-2). All incisions are left open with delayed closure at 2 to 7 days. Split thickness skin grafting is rarely necessary.

Conclusion

Compartment syndrome of the foot is a frequently missed diagnosis. A high index of suspicion for this potential complication of foot trauma is vital, as well as knowledge of the anatomy of the foot in order to diagnose and treat this condition. Expedient release is indicated to avoid long-term sequelae and poor outcomes.

References

1. Perry MD, Manoli A 2nd. Foot compartment syndrome. *Orthop Clin North Am.* 2001;32(1):103-111.
2. Myerson MS. Management of compartment syndromes of the foot. *Clin Orthop Relat Res.* 1991;(271):239-248.
3. Manoli A 2nd, Weber TG. Fasciotomy of the foot: an anatomical study with special reference to release of the calcaneal compartment. *Foot Ankle Int.* 1990;10(5):267-275.
4. Fulkerson E, Razi A, Tejwani N. Acute compartment syndrome of the foot. *Foot Ankle Int.* 2003;24(2):180-187.
5. Mittlmeier T, Machler G, Lob G, Mutschler W, Bauer G, Vogl T. Compartment syndrome of the foot after intraarticular calcaneal fracture. *Clin Orthop Relat Res.* 1991;(269):241-248.

SECTION III

GENERAL FRACTURE CARE

I Have a 38-Year-Old Male in an MVC With Multiple Orthopedic Injuries. Should I Fix Everything Now or Do Damage Control Orthopedics?

Jason W. Nascone, MD
John C. P. Floyd, MD

Damage control is a naval term coined for keeping the vessel afloat and staving off further damage to the ship that can be caused by ignoring the damage already done. Medically, the term may refer to the management of the critically injured patient in a broad sense, or more specifically as a way of temporizing complex orthopedic injuries for staged reconstruction.

Critically injured patients with multiple orthopedic injures present a very complex treatment challenge. These patients cannot be managed in a vacuum. Patients often have a variety of open injuries, fractures, visceral injuries, multiple sources of hemorrhage, and injuries to the neural system. Successful treatment requires close communication between trauma surgeons, orthopedics, and often neurosurgeons. Damage control in this setting refers to halting the ongoing injury. In its basic definition, this means optimizing resuscitation. Correction of hypovolemia, hypothermia, and coagulopathies are paramount for survival. The orthopedic goals in this type of patient consist of controlling hemorrhage, debriding open fractures, and provisional skeletal stabilization. Knowing how much surgery a patient in shock can tolerate can be difficult.[1] Persistent hemodynamic instability or worsening neurologic injury are obvious indicators for damage control techniques. Lactate levels serve as a useful monitor for the level of resuscitation and level of end-organ perfusion. The lactate trend is an indication of whether or not the patient is responding to an intervention. Patients with elevated or increasing lactate levels should be considered candidates for damage control techniques.

The goals in this setting should be well thought out. How will I prep the affected extremities to avoid multiple redraping? What will I do if the patient's condition deteriorates after my debridement? What will be the best order to obtain provisional stabilization of fractures to facilitate mobilization? What can I absolutely *not* treat in a splint? Developing the plan ahead of time lets the surgeon visualize potential pitfalls as well as identify safe bail out points in the event of worsening clinical picture. We initially focus on thorough debridements of all open injuries and stabilization of unstable pelvic ring disruptions. Wounds that can be, are closed; others may require negative pressure dressings or bead pouches. Unstable pelvic ring injuries are stabilized provisionally upon presentation with a binder or sheet. An assessment is made as to whether the patient's resuscitation would benefit from external fixation and/or internal fixation.[2,3] Next, is the patient stable enough (responding to resuscitation and improving) to proceed with internal fixation of long bones (femur, tibia, humerus) or should these fractures be spanned with external fixation? External fixation can be performed rapidly without further substantial surgical exposure and without fluoroscopic image intensification. Length, alignment, and rotation are restored and the patient can be rapidly moved to the ICU setting. If the patient is improving, we prefer to proceed with intramedullary stabilization of femurs and then tibias. Femurs otherwise require traction, which is cumbersome in the ICU setting, and high-energy tibias may be problematic in circumferential dressings. Upper extremities in most settings (except vascular injuries and significant open injuries) can be temporized with splints. During and after each intervention, the patient needs to be assessed as to whether proceeding would be beneficial or detrimental.

Temporizing complex fracture management is also a type of damage control. Complex periarticular fractures, articular fractures, and large soft-tissue wounds may benefit from spanning external fixation upon presentation. The stabilized limb may be elevated from the frame and soft tissues are allowed to recover. The complex injury can then be further imaged and a thoughtful plan developed and executed during daylight hours. Fractures readily amenable to this technique are complex supracondylar femur fractures, complex tibial plateau fractures, pilon fractures, and simple fracture patterns with complex soft-tissue injuries.

Each patient needs to be individualized. Patient status, surgeon status, and injury severity all play an important part in the decision to proceed with damage control orthopedics.

References

1. Roberts CS, Pape HC, Jones AL, Malkani AL, Rodriguez JL, Giannoudis PV. Damage control orthopaedics: evolving concepts in the treatment of patients who have sustained orthopaedic trauma. *Instr Course Lect.* 2005;54:447-462.
2. Nowotarski PJ, Turen CH, Brumback RJ, Scarboro JM. Conversion of external fixation to intramedullary nailing for fractures of the shaft of the femur in multiply injured patients. *J Bone Joint Surg Am.* 2000;82(6):781-788.
3. Scalea TM, Boswell SA, Scott JD, Mitchell KA, Kramer ME, Pollak AN. External fixation as a bridge to intramedullary nailing for patients with multiple injuries and with femur fractures: damage control orthopedics. *J Trauma.* 2000; 48(4):613-623.

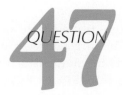

DO BONE STIMULATORS WORK ON NONUNIONS?

Blane Sessions, MD
Craig Castleman Greene, MD

In an effort to advance fracture healing, techniques of internal and external fracture immobilization have been paired with properly timed transmission of physiologic forces across fracture sites. Adjunctive treatment options, such as bone stimulators, have also been used in an attempt to stimulate normal fracture healing in delayed unions and nonunions.

Electric and electromagnetic energy stimulators were devised to treat nonunions based on observations that electric fields occur in mechanically loaded bones.[1] Under mechanical stress, according to Wolff's law, bone remodels in response to piezoelectric charges. The compression side is electronegative, stimulating osteoblasts, which are bone forming, and the tension side is electropositive, stimulating osteoclasts, which are bone resorbing. Artificially promoting these charges with an electric current would therefore theoretically accelerate bone healing. There are three methods in general use—two are considered noninvasive and one invasive.

Electric fields are produced noninvasively using either capacitive coupling (CC) or inductive coupling (IC). In the CC technique, skin electrodes are placed on opposite sides of the fractured bone site with a power source linked to both. IC most commonly uses a pulsed electromagnetic field (PEMF). This technique induces a secondary electrical field in the bone. The induced field is related to the characteristics of the applied apparatus and the biological properties of the bone. Numerous configurations have been studied. Direct electrical current (DC) is utilized through surgically implanted electrodes with the cathode placed in the area of nonunion and the anode being placed in soft tissue nearby. Power sources are then imbedded or place externally.

Clinical studies of delayed unions and nonunions have mostly been centered on using PEMF.[1] A comprehensive review was performed comparing 28 studies of ununited tibial fractures treated with PEMF compared to 14 studies of similar fractures treated with bone graft with or without internal fixation. The overall success rate for the surgical treatment with bone grafting of 569 tibial fractures was 82% (70% to 100%) and by comparison, the overall success rate of PEMF treatment of 1718 tibial fractures was 81% (13% to 100%).[2] Observational studies using invasive DC techniques show rates of union as high as 70% to 90%.[1] The greatest benefit of a bone stimulator may be in multiple bone-grafted non-unions[1] because several reports have shown low success rates in multiple bone-grafted nonunions.[2] One study had successful union rates of 82% using electrical stimulation in 44 patients with multiply grafted tibial nonunions.[3] In this series, 87% of infected fractures healed.

Nonunions, like any other fracture, should be adequately stabilized and have good healing potential (adequate tissue coverage, good blood supply, etc) before considering a stimulator. Delayed or nonunions that are malaligned demand surgical correction before healing can occur, regardless of whether a bone stimulator is used. The presence of a synovial pseudarthrosis in a nonunion is a contraindication to the use of electric stimulation alone.[4] The few randomized controlled studies in delayed and nonunions suggest improved results with electric and electromagnetic fields compared with placebo treatment, and are equivalent to bone grafts.[1]

We prefer the use of external electrical stimulation in nonunions or delayed unions. In order for external stimulation to work, you must have the appropriate length, alignment, and stability of the fracture. We stress to our patients that if we can avoid surgery by the use of an external stimulation device and possibly create the same benefits as that of surgery, it is a very viable option. If the delayed or nonunion does not heal with external stimulation, surgery can then be performed. There is little risk in the application of the external bone stimulator compared to the risk of revision surgery.

References

1. Aaron RK, Ciombor DM, Simon BJ. Treatment of nonunions with electric and electromagnetic fields. *Clin Orthop.* 2004;419:21-29.
2. Gossling HR, Bernstein RA, Abbott J. Treatment of ununited tibial fractures: a comparison of surgery and pulsed electromagnetic fields (PEMF). *Orthopaedics.* 1992;15:711-719.
3. Paterson D, Lewis G, Cass C. Treatment of delayed union and nonunion with an implanted direct current stimulator. *Clin Orthop.* 1980;148:117-128.
4. Nelson FR, Brighton CT, Ryaby J, Simon BJ, Nielson JH, Lorich DG, Bolander M, Seelig J. Use of physical forces in bone healing. *J Am Acad Orthop Surg.* 2003;11:344-354.

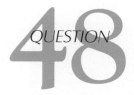
WHEN DO YOU USE LOCKING PLATES?

Thomas F. Higgins, MD

The indications, capabilities, and limitations of nonlocking plate and screw osteo-synthesis have been established and widely taught, most notably through the efforts of the AO/ASIF Group. These tenets were established through study, testing, and several decades of clinical trial-and-error.

Locking plate technology, on the other hand, has been conceived, developed, and rushed to market all within the last 15 years. The result has been widespread confusion about the indications and limitations of this technology. Early experience and judicious employment of these systems may hopefully avoid repeating much of the clinical trial-and-error that taught us so much about nonlocked plating.

The fundamental mechanical weakness in a nonlocked plating construct, properly applied, is toggle between the head of the screw and the plate. This allows movement of the plate relative to the bone, which in turn leads to pullout forces on the screws. Because of the freedom of movement between the screw head and the plate, each screw resists the pullout forces individually. As each screw starts to pull out, the pullout forces placed on the remaining screw heads become more and more concentrated. With locking plate constructs, eliminating the toggle at the screw-plate interface may strengthen the construct at every screw simultaneously. In order for the locked screws to pullout, they would all have to cut through the bone simultaneously, a much higher threshold to be reached by the deforming forces on the construct.

There are some further potential advantages to locking plate systems. Because locking screws are not counting on compression of the plate to the bone for construct stability, this may allow for better preservation of the soft tissues directly over the bone by not having to press the plate up against the bone. The fixed angle between the plate and screw may also permit the use of unicortical screws. With regard to disadvantages, greater compression may be achieved in some instances with regular dynamic compression plates, and

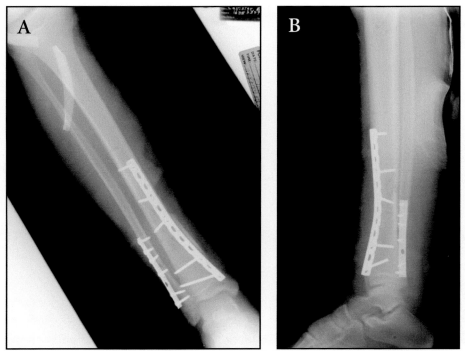

Figure 48-1. Compression plating of simple diaphyseal injuries in healthy bone should not necessitate locking plates.

in most diaphyseal injuries and partial articular injuries, locking plates entail greater expense with no great gain in stability (Figure 48-1). Most "B-type" (partial articular) fractures require only nonlocking buttress fixation, and locking fixation offers no advantage (Figure 48-2).

Translating this into practical applications for open reduction and internal fixation (ORIF), indications for locking plates may be lumped into three broad categories:

1. Fixation of short articular segments to the diaphysis, or periprosthetic fractures

2. Bridging of a diaphyseal or metaphyseal-diaphyseal segment of bone in an effort to minimize soft-tissue dissection and promote callus formation

3. Enhanced fixation in osteoporotic bone

Taking each in turn: With nonlocked fixation, the varus and valgus stresses on the metaphyseal fixation of articular and periarticular fractures may lead to early loss of reduction, and particularly around the knee and proximal humerus, this will occur via varus collapse. Locking plates applied to a reduced metaphyseal and articular segment allow much better resistance to collapse of the opposite cortex and permit less disruption of the soft tissues, thereby promoting healing, often by callus (Figure 48-3). This has been especially helpful in the proximal humerus and distal femur, but there has been much debate on this topic in bicondylar tibial plateau fractures. With a displaced posteromedial or medial fragment, a medial dissection and buttress plating has proven advantageous, proving stronger than isolated lateral locked plate fixation. Periprosthetic fractures are analogous to a short articular segment, and locking fixation has been an important addition to the treatment of these injuries (Figure 48-4).

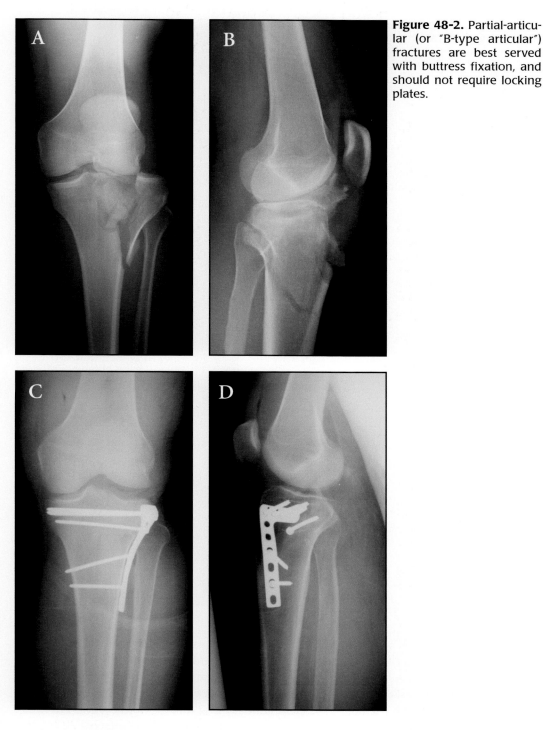

Figure 48-2. Partial-articular (or "B-type articular") fractures are best served with buttress fixation, and should not require locking plates.

"Bridging" of long segments with locking fixation promotes minimal soft-tissue disruption and encourages callus formation. This has been used to permit submuscular plating and percutaneous techniques. However, this may be more demanding than open

Figure 48-3. "Bridging" locked fixation yields callus healing, much like an intramedullary nail.

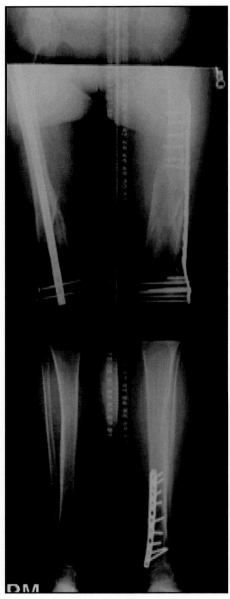

techniques because the surgeon must judge, indirectly or fluoroscopically, the correct achievement of length, rotation, and alignment of the limb. In some of these percutaneous techniques, as well as in some uses of open locked plating, unicortical locking screws may be used in diaphyseal segments. A bridging technique applied with the locking plate not placed firmly against the bone will yield bone healing though callus, similar to intermedulllary nails or external fixation, and has thus yielded the term "internal ex-fix" for locking fixation in some settings (see Figure 48-3). Percutaneous or minimally invasive fixation techniques may be facilitated by locking implants because they do not require as much direct opposition to the underlying bone (Figure 48-5).

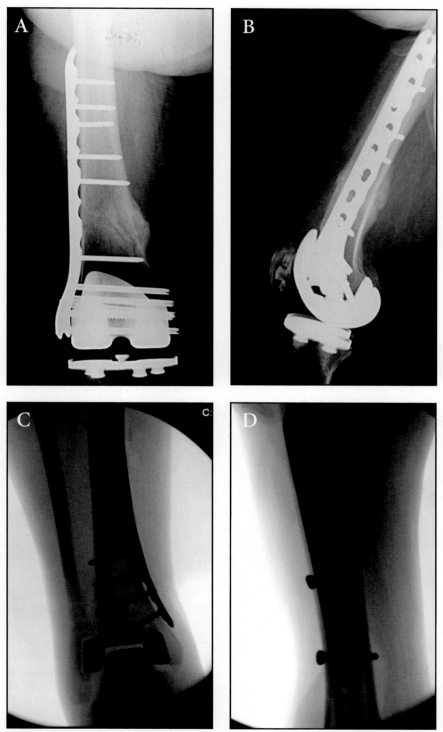

Figure 48-4. Periprosthetic fractures may behave like short articular segments (containing a prosthesis). This is often a good indication for locked plate fixation.

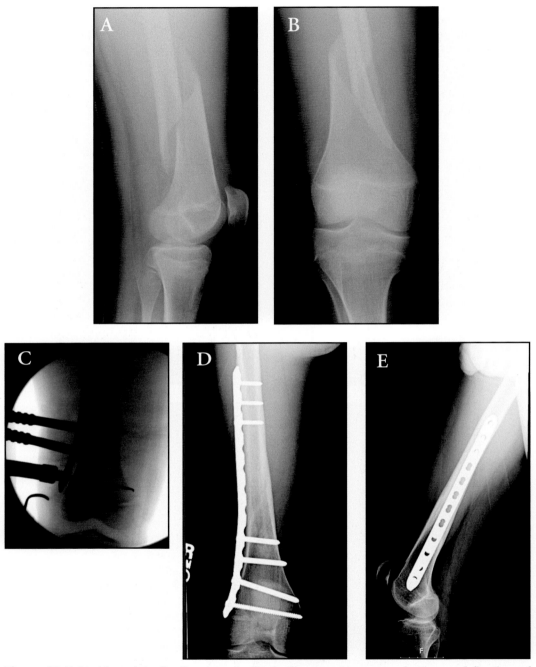

Figure 48-5. Locking plate fixation may facilitate the percutaneous reduction and fixation of metaphyseal or diaphyseal injuries, as illustrated by this 15-year-old male with open physes and a femur fracture. Submuscular plating was achieved through two incisions, with a non-locked screw used distally to avoid the physis.

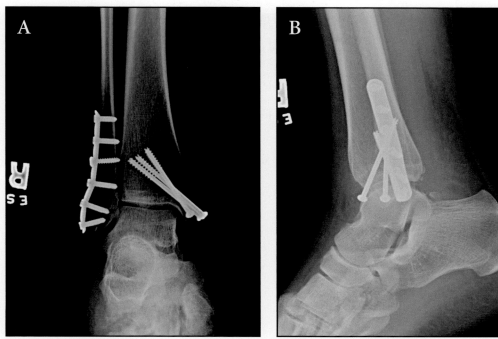

Figure 48-6. This application of locking fixation in healthy bone adds little value and increases costs in a setting where a non-locking posterolateral anti-glide would perform admirably.

The enhanced fixation achieved in osteoporotic bone is certainly an advance from previous technology, but is by no means a panacea. Using locking fixation in osteoporotic bone will not magically guarantee purchase, and in some cases may simply deny the surgeon any tactile feedback as to how poor the bone is. Nonetheless, elimination of the toggle at the screw-plate interface has been shown to offer enhanced resistance to failure in osteoporotic bone. However, in a fracture scenario where one might otherwise use uni-cortical locking screws in healthy bone, bicortical locking screws may still be advisable in the osteoporotic patient.

Conclusion

Locked plating is certainly one method to improve the stability of the bone and plate construct, but is not indicated in all settings, and by no means replaces non-locked plating (Figure 48-6). While the three indications listed above may serve as guidelines, under-standing the goals of a given fracture surgery and employing good soft-tissue technique are probably more important than the type of fixation used.

Bibliography

1. Wagner M. General principles for the clinical use of the LCP. *Injury.* 2003;34 Suppl 2:B31-42.
2. Greiwe RM, Archdeacon MT. Locking plate technology: current concepts. *J Knee Surg.* 2007;20(1):50-5.
3. Higgins TF, Klatt J, Bachus KN. Biomechanical analysis of bicondylar tibial plateau fixation: how does lateral locking plate fixation compare to dual plate fixation? *J Orthop Trauma.* 2007;21(5):301-6.
4. Haidukewych GJ. Innovations in locking plate technology. *J Am Acad Orthop Surg.* 2004;12(4):205-12.
5. Gardner MJ, Helfet DL, Lorich DG. Has locked plating completely replaced conventional plating? *Am J Orthop.* 2004;33(9):439-46.

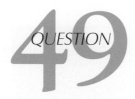
WHICH FRACTURES REQUIRE ANATOMIC REDUCTION?

Medardo Marota, MD
Walter W. Virkus, MD

While traditional recommendations for fracture treatment are *anatomic reduction* and *rigid fixation*, these principles have evolved recently to *adequate reduction* and *stable fixation*. These changes have evolved from the experience that anatomic reduction of some fractures leads to excessive soft-tissue stripping and devascularization. The concentration on adequate reduction and stable fixation shifts the focus on some fractures to restoration of length, alignment and rotation, without the need for anatomic reduction of multiple fracture fragments. The adequacy of the reduction required is determined by the fracture location and amount of comminution. The type of reduction must be matched with the appropriate type of stability and fixation. Stability can be either absolute or relative.

Relative stability allows a small amount of fracture displacement between fracture fragments when load is applied. This interfragmentary motion stimulates secondary bone healing via callus formation. Excess motion at the fracture site due to insufficient stability may lead to nonunion, usually a hypertrophic nonunion. Common methods of obtaining relative stability include casting, external fixation, intramedullary nailing, and bridge plating, in increasing order of stability.

Absolute stability is achieved when interfragmentary motion is eliminated, which allows primary bone healing to occur by direct bone remodeling. No callus is seen in primary bone healing. Absolute stability is obtained by direct fracture compression, which can be obtained with a lag screw or compression plating. Lag screw compression is weak in torsional loading, and therefore must be combined with a neutralization plate (Figure 49-1). Absolute stability requires an anatomic reduction. Callus will not form in the presence of absolute stability, so if significant gaps exist after reduction, they will persist and nonunion will result. In this situation, the nonunion is usually atrophic.

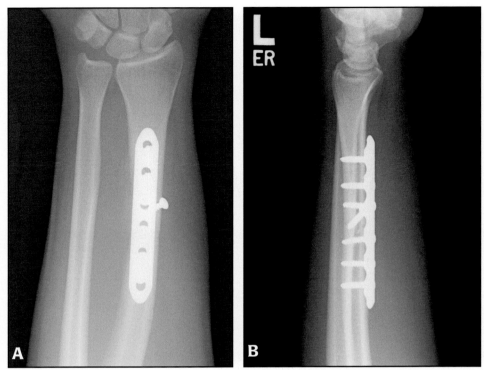

Figure 49-1. AP (A) and lateral (B) radiograph of a radial shaft fracture with lag screws and compression plate. Absolute stability in a radial shaft fracture using interfragmentary lag screws and compression plating. Note the absence of callus formation.

While anatomic reduction and absolute stability sounds optimal, this often requires extensive exposure, subperiosteal stripping, liberal use of circumferential clamps, multiple lag screws, and compression plates. These techniques devascularize fracture fragments and increase the chance of nonunion and infection in comminuted fractures. Therefore, we reserve anatomic reduction for articular fractures and simple forearm fractures. We stabilize our anatomic reductions with a lag screw whenever possible, and with compression plating in tranverse fractures where a lag screw is not possible. Although most long bone diaphyseal fractures heal well with relative stability, diaphyseal fractures of the forearm are an exception. The small diameter of the radius and ulna, and resultant small fracture area of simple fractures, leads to unreliable healing with relative stability.

We treat the majority of nonarticular fractures using a more biologically friendly approach, including closed or minimally open reduction and relative stability with intramedullary nailing or bridge plating. We focus on restoring anatomically correct length, mechanical axis alignment, and proper rotation. We essentially ignore multiple small fracture fragments between the two articular segments of the injured bone, concentrating on overall alignment. We use intramedullary fixation for diaphyseal fractures. For metaphyseal fractures, bridge plating has become more common, with either open or percutaneous placement of the plate and screws. Similar to intramedullary nailing, the

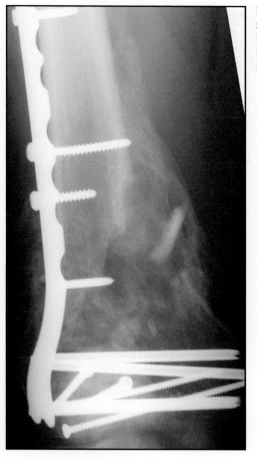

Figure 49-2. Combined relative and absolute stability in a severely comminuted supracondylar/intracondylar distal femur fracture. Note the presence of callus formation in the metaphyseal region.

reduction focuses on length, alignment, and rotation. Bridge plates act as internal splints spanning areas of comminution. These plates are affixed only to the major proximal and distal fracture fragments and no interfragmentary compression occurs. Thus, comminuted fragments remain untouched and retain their soft-tissue attachments, allowing secondary healing by callus.

Some fractures are best treated with a combination of anatomic and nonanatomic reduction with absolute and relative stability. Articular fractures with metaphyseal comminution, such as the tibial plateau and distal femur, are common examples. In these cases, we reduce the articular component of these fractures anatomically and stabilize them with lag screws. This is typically performed through a relatively small incision near the joint surface. We then align the metaphyseal and diaphyseal components using a closed reduction technique such as a femoral distractor, and apply a plate to bridge the fracture area with fixation in the articular segment adjacent to the articular lag screws, and on the opposite side of the fracture in the diaphysis. This allows secondary healing with callus of this comminuted segment. Implants such as locking plates can be used to facilitate this bridge plating construct, particularly if the end segments are short or the bone is poor quality (Figure 49-2).

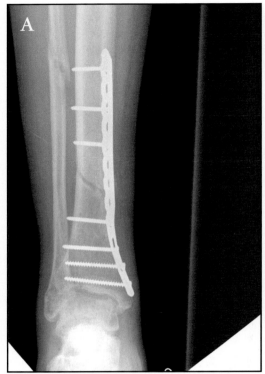 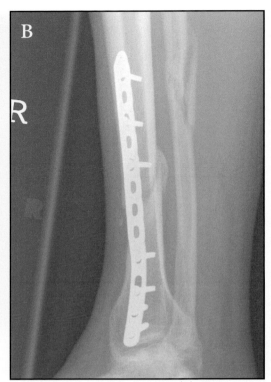

Figure 49-3. Relative stability with bridge plating of a spiral distal tibia fracture (A). Note posterior callus on lateral radiograph (B).

Lastly, some fractures can be treated with either anatomic reduction and absolute stability, or nonanatomic reduction and relative stability. We see this scenario in metaphyseal fractures with a single transverse, spiral, or oblique fracture line (Figures 49-3 and 49-4). In these cases, our treatment will be directed by the status of the soft tissue, with a tenuous soft-tissue envelope directing us toward a closed reduction and relative stability with either a plate or an intramedullary nail. If a plate is used, a lag screw should not be placed across the fracture if an anatomic reduction is not obtained. The plate construct should be stabilized, leaving one or two screw holes on each side of the fracture unfilled to allow a small amount of motion at the fracture site, which will lead to secondary healing with callus.

References

1. Shatzker J, Tile M. *The Rationale of Operative Fracture Care.* 3rd ed. Berlin: Springer-Verlag; 2005.
2. Ruedi TP, Murphy WM. *AO Principles of Fracture Management.* New York: AO Publishing Thieme; 2000.
3. Leunig M, Hertel R, Siebenrock KA, Ballmer FT, Mast, JW, Ganz R. The evolution of indirect reduction techniques for the treatment of fractures. *Clin Orthop Relat Res.* 2000. 375:7-14.

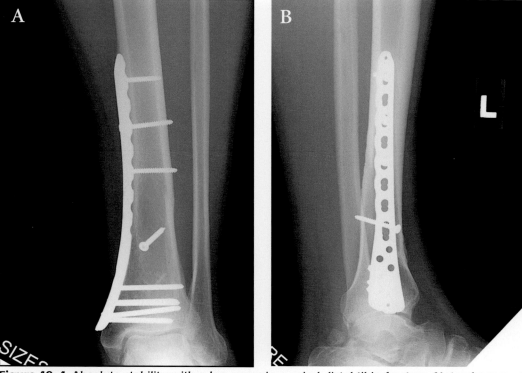

Figure 49-4. Absolute stability with a lag screw in a spiral distal tibia fracture. Note absence of callus.

INDEX

Printed in the United States
by Baker & Taylor Publisher Services